PENGUIN BOOKS

HELP FOR THE OVERWEIGHT CHILD

Jurgen M. Wolff is a se
ing Achievement Corp
is also associated with

Dr. Dewey Lipe is a
Schools, and this book is based on the successful program
of the schools in Los Altos, California. He is affiliated
with American Institutes for Research and with Behavior
Therapy Associates. He is coauthor with Jurgen M. Wolff
of a diet book for adults, *Slimmanship*.

Help for the Overweight Child

Jurgen M. Wolff
and
Dewey Lipe, Ph.D.

PENGUIN BOOKS

Penguin Books Ltd, Harmondsworth,
Middlesex, England
Penguin Books, 625 Madison Avenue,
New York, New York 10022, U.S.A.
Penguin Books Australia Ltd, Ringwood,
Victoria, Australia
Penguin Books Canada Limited, 2801 John Street,
Markham, Ontario, Canada L3R 1B4
Penguin Books (N.Z.) Ltd, 182–190 Wairau Road,
Auckland 10, New Zealand

First published in the United States of America by
Stein and Day/*Publishers* 1978
Published in Penguin Books 1980

LIBRARY OF CONGRESS CATALOGING IN PUBLICATION DATA
Wolff, Jurgen.
Help for the overweight child.
1. Obesity in children. 2. Reducing. I. Lipe,
Dewey, joint author. II. Title.
[RJ399.c6w64 1980]   618.9′23′98   79–21795
ISBN 0 14 00.5318 2

Printed in the United States of America by
Offset Paperback Mfrs., Inc., Dallas, Pennsylvania
Set in Caledonia

Contents

Introduction

"Hey kid, how come you're so fat?" To some people that sounds like a funny question. The one person for whom it isn't funny is the child on the receiving end. Maybe your boy or girl has come running home in tears after hearing this kind of question; or maybe you just want to make sure it's a question your child never has to hear. Either way, this book will help.

The fact that you're reading this book shows that you recognize how important it is to keep your child's weight at the right level. Frankly, you're miles ahead of most parents. Most mothers and fathers make sure their children have the newest Bionic Megacharged Realistic Supertoy (batteries not included). They buy them the latest in flared, faded, or updated clothes. They try to help out when junior gets lost in the new math or the old math or the middle-aged math. But a lot of times they don't give much thought to their children's weight. How often have you heard comments like these:

"Babies should be chubby. It's a sign of good health."

"That's just baby fat, nothing to worry about."

"Chubby kids are happy that way. If you try to get them to lose weight, you make them grow up too fast."

All of these statements are wrong. Chubbiness is not a sign of good health, not in adults and not in babies. When a child is fat, it *is* something to worry about. A fat child is likely to become a fat adult. An overweight adult is less healthy than a slimmer adult. The longer you wait to correct a child's weight problem, the harder it is. Also, an obese child is usually unhappy. An overweight child is different, and being different is a cardinal sin among kids. The fat child is unmercifully teased and left out of activities. Helping your child to be trimmer doesn't make him or her grow up too fast—it liberates your child. It increases the chances that your child's adolescence and adulthood will be free of physical and emotional problems.

This book is a workbook. First it tells you the facts you need to know about the causes and penalties of being overweight, about nutrition and exercise, about the psychology of weight loss, and about other subjects relating to eating and weight control. Then it shows you, step-by-step, how to give your children good eating and exercise habits to make them slimmer, healthier, and happier. This book isn't too long and it doesn't contain a lot of technical language or theory, nor does it contain a magic formula to instantly melt the fat off your child's body. But it does contain advice and a plan that works. It is based on the successful experience of clients of the Self-Management Schools in Los Altos, California, and it builds on the foundation of our weight-control book for adults, *Slimmanship.*

Chapter by chapter, here's what you'll find in *Help for the Overweight Child:*

Chapter One reveals the penalties of being an overweight child. Some of the penalties are obvious, some are equally serious but hidden. If you still have doubts about whether a weight-control program for your child is worth the effort, this chapter will convince you. It will also help you explain the program to your boy or girl and enlist his or her cooperation.

Chapter Two tells you why your child is overweight. It shows you that your child is far from alone in having this problem, and it gives you a guide to desirable weight levels for children of various ages, heights, and builds.

Chapter Three discusses nutrition. You don't have to put on a white smock and turn your kitchen into a lab. It doesn't even matter if you flunked biology and chemistry—all you need are some basic facts about the four food groups and how to give your child a balanced diet. It's also important that you understand some of the myths about nutrition, myths spread by advertisers.

Chapter Four follows up with important information about the other main weapon used to attack obesity: exercise. It includes a chart showing how many calories are used up by different types of exercise. You'll find out what's the best exercise for kids, how you can encourage your children to be more active, and how to enlist the help of your child's physical education teacher.

Chapter Five describes the ten most important eating-related behaviors. You'll probably find that your boy or girl has been having trouble with several of these behaviors. Now you'll see there are good alternatives to every bad eating habit your child has developed.

Naturally, reading about an alternative and getting your child to go along with it are two different things. But eating is a behavior just like any other behavior. Children are born with the need for food, but they learn (mostly from their parents) where, what, when, and how much to eat. Chapter Six reveals the psychological tools you can use to change your child's eating habits. The key to changing behavior is using incentives (rewards), and Chapter Six also explains what incentives are, how they can be applied, and provides successful case studies. You'll find that rewards need not be physical things like toys or money—the best incentives are free.

Chapter Seven recommends specific incentives you can use with your child. It discusses how different rewards are required at different age levels and shows how you can gradually phase out rewards once a behavior has been changed.

Chapter Eight is the most important part of the book. At this point you stop reading and start acting. Using the information you will have picked up from the other chapters, you design a weight-loss and weight-control program that fits the needs of your child. You will pick a weight goal, choose the problems to attack first, and select the incentives you will use to get the results you want. There are charts that make this an easy job and a calendar to help you keep track of your child's progress.

The last chapter will come in handy once your child has reached his or her ideal weight. It is concerned with *keeping* your child trim. The system explained in this book is not based on fads or gimmicks; so once good eating and exercise habits are established they are relatively simple to keep up. Chapter Nine describes how to do it—it alerts you to the weight dangers to watch for as your child enters adolescence, tells how to change incentives as your boy or girl gets older, and how to use reminder incentives when necessary.

We've also supplied two useful appendices: One tells you how many calories there are in most common foods, and the other provides recipes for healthful snacks for children of all ages.

The best way to begin is to begin. Turn now to Chapter One, and you'll be moving closer to the day when your child no longer has to endure the painful question, "Hey kid, how come you're so fat?"

Jurgen Wolff
Dewey Lipe

Help for the Overweight Child

1

The World of the Overweight Child

The overweight child pays a price for his or her condition. It's almost as if every extra pound adds another penalty. These penalties come in various forms: social, psychological, and physical. Let's take a look at the world of the fat child and the punishment that's a part of that world.

Social Penalties

Adults tend to think of childhood as a carefree time, full of fun and loyal playmates. It's partly due to poor memories and partly to wishful thinking. We like to forget childhood's cruel side. Whether or not they mean to hurt each other, kids can be very clever at finding each other's weak spots and exploiting them. Children soon learn that there are certain qualities that supposedly go with being fat. Fat people are piggy, they're lazy, and they're jokers. Think back to your own days at school. Most likely you'll remember that there was at least one fat kid in the group, and he or she wasn't treated quite the same by the other children. Where do kids get these mistaken ideas? Mostly from their parents and other adults. The same people who compliment you for having a chubby baby or a roly-poly five year old assume that fat adolescents and adults must be weak or slothful or jolly.

Children also make fun of their fat friends for "looking funny." Not only are they large, they wear "funny clothes." A dress designed for a sixteen-year-old girl, cut down to fit a ten year old, does look strange. So does a twelve-year-old boy wearing his father's altered sports jacket.

So it's not surprising that being overweight can lead to social isolation. The kid who's nicknamed "Fatso" or "Piggy" is seldom popular as a friend, seldom picked for athletic contests, seldom invited to social events.

The child who is left out usually figures out a way to compensate, a way to fit in with the crowd. As discussed in the next part of this chapter, these compensations are not always good for the child. Sometimes he will be very self-critical to show the other kids he realizes he's different and he's willing to associate with them as an inferior rather than as an equal. Whatever form this kind of compensatory behavior takes, it can interfere with normal social development.

The heaviest social penalties for being overweight occur during adolescence. It's already a confusing time when sexual awareness increases and when a premium is put upon how you look. Teenagers of both sexes spend hours of effort and lots of money to make sure that their clothes, hair, complexion, breath, and smell are as desirable as possible. Body odor can be washed away, mouth washes can get rid of bad breath, creams can cover up pimples, shampoos and cream rinses can fix split ends, and an infusion of allowance money keeps wardrobes up-to-date. But there's no easy solution to being 30 pounds overweight.

All too often, fat boys are too self-conscious to ask for dates, and fat girls aren't asked. Both sit around alone on Friday and Saturday nights. Ideally, members of the opposite sex would notice what a great personality your son or daughter has and not worry about his or her weight. Too bad it doesn't happen that way. For the fat teenager, the growing-up years are lonely and bitter.

Some of the obvious social discrimination against overweight people stops when they grow up. Seldom will anyone call them fatso anymore, at least not to their face. After all, if you're big you may pack a hefty punch or swing a mean handbag. But overweight adults do encounter problems: Clothes still will never fit quite right, some people will still assume that to be overweight is to be lazy and weak willed, and overweight people will even be discriminated against when it comes to job promotions. So it's not safe to assume that the social penalties of obesity will end when the child grows up.

Psychological Penalties

A child starts life with no way of defining itself. A baby doesn't know who he or she is. That definition is provided by others: first by parents and relatives, then by teachers and other children. Analysis of children's behavior indicates that they believe the labels applied to them, and they mold their behavior to fit the labels.

Let's look at an example of how this works. Ralph D. is a construction worker who prides himself on his strength and courage. He was very happy when his second child was a boy. But Ralph was disturbed that Jimmy (unlike Beth, his older sister) cried a lot as a baby. Almost from the start, Ralph considered Jimmy a "cry baby" and called him that whenever Jimmy reacted to a problem with tears. Gradually the message, "I am a cry baby," worked its way into Jimmy's mind. You have probably noticed that there's a pause between a problem and a child's reaction to it. When a knee has been skinned, the child seems to stop for a second to decide whether to scream, sniffle, or kick the ground to get even. During these moments of decision, Jimmy's subconscious reminded him that he was a cry baby and that the way a cry baby reacts to problems is by bursting into tears. So that's what he did, and of course the cycle was completed when his father again called him a cry baby.

The same kind of thing happens with overweight children. If being fat didn't have so many bad associations, this wouldn't be a problem. People would say, "You're overweight," the child would realize "I'm overweight," and it would end there. But as we have already seen, when someone says, "You're overweight," he is also often saying "You're lazy, piggy, and socially undesirable." If the child internalizes this information, he or she then may *act* lazy, piggy, and socially undesirable and close the circle by conforming to what other people expect.

Not all adults are so unkind in their attitudes. Some are very sympathetic, but then the sympathy turns into pity. The fat child gets used to hearing, or overhearing, comments like this:

"That poor girl, I don't know what will ever become of her. I certainly don't think she'll be able to find a husband."

"It's funny, all of Bobby's brothers and sisters are normal. I wonder how come he's so overweight."

"Too bad about Linda. And she has such a pretty face!"

Even the young child knows that pity is reserved for the weak, the ugly, the unfortunate. He or she is likely to withdraw from the well-intentioned pitying looks that are all around.

Feelings of inferiority also affect what children expect from the future. Children start out feeling that they can be anything they want to be. They build fantasies about being a fire-fighter, a stewardess, a pilot, a model, a professional ball player. Overweight children start life feeling restricted: How many fat fire-fighters, stewardesses, or pilots have they ever seen?

As briefly mentioned before, children who feel inferior generally find a way to make up for these feelings. Once in a while this compensation can be constructive. For example, a child who is not athletic may make an extra effort to do well in academic work. At other times, the compensatory activity is negative. The child may try to be popular in spite of being overweight by becoming the class joker, the most daring in the group, or the first to defy authority. As well as leading to psychological problems by making the child feel that he continually has to prove himself, this naturally can lead to behavior problems.

The overweight child who starts out with supportive parents may have developed a strong, self-confident image by the time he or she comes into contact with other children. This kind of child will be better able to cope with criticism or insults from others, but can still react by becoming a loner and resenting the stereotype with which he or she is saddled.

All this is not to say that it is impossible for an overweight child to grow up to be a well-adjusted, happy adult. But it is true that the overweight child starts out with a strike against him or her and will have to work harder at the already difficult task of growing up.

Physical Penalties

The health hazards of being overweight are well known. The more extreme the obesity, the harder the heart has to work and the more likely it is that the individual will suffer heart disease. Here are some of the other physical problems that more often bother the overweight person than the slim person:

diabetes
arthritis
high blood pressure
varicose veins
kidney disease
constipation
inflammation of the gall bladder
for women, problems during pregnancy and childbirth

These problems won't show up during childhood, but during these formative years the scene is set for them. It's no good assuming that the fat child will automatically grow out of his or her weight problem, or that a little exercise will solve everything. Since the fat child isn't good at games that require speed and agility, he or she will avoid exercise. Being a social loner adds to this— few kids go bowling alone or hiking alone. So the overweight child forms a partnership with the TV screen and the chocolate bar, and the weight problem gets worse instead of better. Increased flabbiness and loss of muscle tone then are added to the other physical penalties.

Your Child's World

What you have read so far may scare you, but that's not our purpose. We are trying to point out how great a change for the better you can make in your child's life by helping him or her to reduce. The campaign outlined in this book will not always be easy. The same can be said of taking a child to the dentist, but you do it anyway because you understand what will happen if you don't. In the same way, you now understand the possible results of not making the effort to help your child become slim. It's a commitment you, the parent, have to make because your child is too young to do it.

To see how being overweight is already affecting *your* child, take a couple of minutes to fill in the Penalties charts.

On the page headlined "Social Penalties," jot down specific examples of times when your boy or girl has been left out because he or she is overweight. You don't have to write a long description of each incident—if your daughter wasn't invited to a party, just jot down "missed out on party," if you heard some kids call your boy an unkind nickname, write down the nickname. Think back and list as many examples as you can.

On the page headlined "Psychological Penalties," indicate examples of how your child has shown some psychological problems as a result of being obese. Has he asked why he's different from the other kids? Has your daughter been depressed after being teased? Again, list several specific examples.

Finally, on the page headlined "Physical Penalties," list examples of how being overweight has affected the health or physical performance of your child. Again, the serious diseases associated with obesity don't tend to show up until adulthood, but you may find that your child is out of breath after running short distances, or that he or she gets bad grades in physical education.

Some people hesitate to write in a book—please don't hesitate. This is a workbook, and it's designed so you can write all sorts of information in it. There are two reasons for having you fill in these particular charts. The first is to demonstrate that what is important isn't the theory of obesity or how it has affected people in our case studies, but rather the effect it is having on your own child. The second purpose is to motivate you to follow through with your efforts. If you ever get bored or frustrated with the process of changing your child's behavior (and his or her weight), look back at these charts and you'll be reconvinced that it's worth the effort.

SOCIAL PENALTIES

PSYCHOLOGICAL PENALTIES

PHYSICAL PENALTIES

What to Tell Your Child

The remaining chapters of this book will give you the tools with which to help your child reduce. You'll learn how to use a system of rewards, also called an incentives structure, that will shape your child's behavior. You can do this without explaining to your child what you're up to, and this is fine if the child is quite young. But if the child is old enough to understand, you can discuss the situation. In these discussions, there are several points to remember:

1) Don't give the child the impression that you are trying to cure a disease or change something terrible into something good. This kind of approach only convinces the child that he or she is a failure. The penalties of obesity listed in this chapter need not be described to the child; rather, stress the benefits of being slim. For example, if the child asks, "But why should I lose weight?" you can simply say, "Because you'll feel better." Obviously, the older the child, the more sophisticated you can be in your explanation.

2) Don't argue about the benefits of losing weight. If the child disagrees with you or insists that he or she doesn't want to lose weight, drop the subject but continue the program. It's a natural tendency to resist change. For example, psychiatrists find that people who are deeply depressed may still cling to that condition because they know what it's like, while the idea of *not* being depressed is frightening

—they don't know whether they'll be able to handle it. Similarly, a fat child may not be happy being called "Fatso," but he may prefer it to the uncertainty of what could happen when he's slimmed down. Eventually the benefits of being slimmer will become apparent to the child simply because he or she will begin experiencing them (but don't rub it in, even then).

3) Don't make a big deal out of the effort. This will only make the child more self-conscious and may cause guilt feelings when there are pauses in progress. As we will explain later, the weight-loss pattern includes times when weight stays the same for a while before going further down. This is hard for kids to understand; so don't involve them in discussion of day-to-day progress. Also, when figuring calories or filling in the calendar charts you'll find later in the book, do so without pointing out to your child that all this effort is going on because of him or her. In fact, some of the things suggested will help improve the health of the whole family, and it's better to stress this when you discuss the changes you're making.

4) Take your cue from your child. If he or she gradually becomes more interested, in a positive way, in what's going on, you can share some of the information you've picked up about nutrition and exercise. You can accomplish your goal with or without the knowing cooperation of your child. Accept and encourage cooperation to the extent your child is ready to offer it.

5) Don't expect (or lead your child to expect) instant

results. If your boy or girl is quite a bit overweight, that condition took a long time to develop, and it will take some time to change. There are gimmicky diets available that lead to quick weight loss. Some of them are hazardous to health, and they bring only temporary benefits. Our approach is a healthy long-term approach.

With these points in mind, you're ready to begin. The next few chapters give you all the information you'll need, starting with a brief discussion of why your child is overweight and the desirable weight levels for children of various ages, heights, and builds.

Chapter Summary

The overweight child pays social, physical, and psychological penalties for weighing too much. He or she is more likely to be a social outcast and as a result may be lonely and have a negative self-image. Most overweight children become overweight adults, and they are then more vulnerable to a variety of diseases and to further social discrimination.

When you begin your efforts to improve your child's eating and exercise habits, it's important not to expect instant results and not to give the child the impression that these efforts are a lot of trouble. Tell your child only as much as he or she wants to know about what you're doing, and don't let yourself be drawn into arguments—some children fear change of any kind, but you can go ahead knowing that you're doing what is best for your child's physical and mental health.

2

Why Your Child Is Fat

Before you can help your child, you have to find out why he or she is overweight. Here are the most common reasons offered by parents:

"My child must have a glandular problem."

It is true that a number of glands affect the growth and weight of children. The one most often referred to as the culprit responsible for obesity is the thyroid gland. It releases hormones that speed up your metabolism (the process by which your body converts food into fuel for its needs). If you have too little of the thyroid hormone, your body doesn't convert food quickly enough and instead stores it as fat. It is sometimes possible to cope with this by reducing the intake of food. Over half the people who have a thyroid hormone deficiency are not overweight.

Only a very small percentage of people—children or adults—have any glandular problems. Even so, before anyone begins an effort to reduce, he or she should see a doctor. The approach we describe in this book is not strenuous, it will not cause any distress to a healthy child.

But you should check with your family doctor to ensure that your boy or girl is healthy and not one of that tiny minority whose weight problems are due to medical factors. We also invite you to discuss our approach with your child's doctor; unlike many fad diets or extreme measures, our approach is based on principles of nutrition and exercise that are accepted by the medical profession.

"Overweight runs in our family. It must be a hereditary problem."

Being overweight may be common in your family, but that doesn't mean it is necessarily a hereditary problem. Heredity refers to traits or characteristics that are passed on in the genes. Although there are exceptions, if both parents have blue eyes, the child is likely to have blue eyes. Similarly, tall children are likely to come from tall families. These sorts of characteristics are permanent and out of our control. It's tempting to dismiss the problem of obesity and say it's out of our control, too. But we also pass on our beliefs and habits to our children. You may know a family in which the grandparents, the parents, and the children all are Republicans, yet you wouldn't say this was due to heredity. Any one of the family members could decide at any time (perhaps at some risk) to become a Democrat.

Beliefs about which foods are good, the idea that you must always finish what's on your plate: these ideas, too, can be passed on from generation to generation. If mother and father are hearty eaters who enjoy lots of snacks while watching television, son or daughter will undoubtedly learn to munch along happily. Even if daughter marries a relative lightweight but she's packing along Mom's recipes, the lightweight will soon be wondering why his trousers don't seem to fit as well as they used to. By the same token, a slim wife may hear demands from her pudgy husband for "great cakes like Mom used to bake." When children come along, they are swept up in the tide of calories. This, rather than heredity, is likely to account for the fact that in 75 percent of the cases in which parents are overweight, the children are overweight. In only 9 percent of the cases in which neither of the parents are overweight do the kids become overweight.

"My kid's fatness is just a phase of growing up."

Being overweight is likely to be the longest phase your child will go through unless something is done to interrupt it. Dr. Alvin B. Hayes, a pediatrician at the Mayo Clinic, has estimated that about 80 percent of overweight children tend to carry their obesity on to adult life. It's true that there will be some variation in weight as children grow up. We are not suggesting that you attempt to control your child's weight down to the ounce or even to the single pound. Any parent who is honest with himself or herself can tell the difference between a child who has reached a plateau where the progress of weight has slightly exceeded the progress of height, and a child who is just plain overweight.

"My child is overweight because he eats too much, or eats the wrong kind of food. Also, he doesn't get enough exercise."

That's a quote from the honest parent who has run out of excuses. Chapter Three will deal in detail with calories and nutrition, but let's take a very quick look at how what you eat affects your weight. To make it simple, food can be compared to fuel. A calorie is, in essence, a unit of fuel. When you're eating the right amount and the right kind of food, you keep your body in good running condition. When you eat too much, your body converts the extra food into fat and stores it by attaching it to various parts of your anatomy. A little reserve fuel is fine; you may need it in an emergency. Overweight people have too many reserves and too few emergencies.

There are two ways, and only two ways, of sensibly reducing body weight. One is to reduce the fuel, so that the body has to use up some of the reserves. This means that you must consume fewer calories. The other way is to keep eating the same amount, but increasing the body's demand for fuel by getting more exercise.

Different kinds of foods have different numbers of calories per ounce. For example, an ounce of chocolate has many more calories than an ounce of carrots. Also, foods vary quite a lot in how nutritious they are. For these reasons, *what* you eat is as important as how much you eat.

So the reason that your child is overweight is that he or she eats too much or eats the wrong kind of food and gets too little exercise. But why is this the case? Parents have to take ultimate responsibility for their children, but there is a villain who has invaded homes and undermined the good intentions of many parents. His name: Television. The passive practice of watching television has replaced many more active pursuits. Perhaps even worse, television advertising is the source of much misinformation about food.

Misinformation about Food

Let's look at some aspects of the relationship between television and children. A study by a University of Pennsylvania student indicates that professionals in the fields of law, pediatrics, and psychiatry feel that television ads may pose a danger to children. Among the findings of this survey of 158 professionals are these:

Of all the mass media, TV has the most powerful effects on children.

Younger kids often can't tell the difference between a TV show and the ads it contains.

TV ads lead children to demand that their parents buy products the parents don't want to buy.

The advertising world recognizes the effect TV has on children. Here's a quote from Jerry Rigglein of Oscar Meyer, and Company, from the July 19, 1965, issue of *Advertising Age* (subsequently, advertisers have become a bit less outspoken, perhaps because they know that consumer advocates are listening in):

When you sell a woman on a product and she goes into the store and finds your brand isn't in stock, she'll probably forget about it. But when you sell a kid on your product, if he can't get it, he will throw himself on the floor, stamp his feet and cry. You can't get a reaction like that out of an adult.

Having established the power of television, let's examine what kids see. On a recent Saturday morning network show, they could have seen up to 24 ads in one hour. Most of the ads were for sugared candies, snacks, and cereals. Probably none of them were for foods recognized to be nutritionally valuable.

In 1973, representatives of Action for Children's Television gave testimony to the U.S. Senate Select Committee on Nutrition and Human Needs on the issue of advertising oversugared foods on children's television. The American Academy of Pediatrics later published a summary of the testimony in their monthly publication. Here are some of the major points:

Food advertising directed to children sets up a conflict between the parent and child and between the child and authority figures such as doctors, dentists, and teachers.

The products sold to children over television are dominated by the four most cavity-producing groups of foods: caramel, chocolate, cookies, and pastry.

Food products advertised on television are more frequently requested by the child than other products.

The food habit promoted by television ads aimed at children teaches that one eats because it's fun, it's sweet, or it's the way to get a premium rather than because it's necessary to good health.

The testimony concluded that television is a medium that could be a powerful educational tool to inform the

American public of good health and nutrition. Instead, it's a vehicle for falsehood, misinformation, and misleading persuasion.

Things are improving a bit. Ads that tell children to ask their parents to buy a specific product have been taken off the air. Cereal ads are beginning to mention nutrition. And the ABC network has been running 30- and 60-second public service announcements giving a little equal time to green beans, cauliflower, and celery.

Even so, many products designed for children are unbelievably loaded with sugar. According to figures released by the Center for Science in the Public Interest in Washington, D.C., Apple Jacks, Fruit Loops, and Sugar Smacks each contained more than 50 percent sugar; Cocoa Krispies contained 46 percent sugar; Sugar Frosted Flakes contained 42 percent, and Sugar Pops and Frosted Rice each contained 39 percent sugar.

Under pressure, the Kellogg Company agreed to put on its packages the amount of sugar each of its cereals contains. But instead of expressing it in percentages, they decided to put it in terms of "grams per ounce," a quantification that will puzzle most buyers. A Kellogg's public relations director declared, "we believe that nobody really cares about the sugar 'non-issue.'"

As you can see, it's up to you to care if you don't want television ads to further contribute to your child's weight problem. Our chapter on nutrition will tell you more about the myths pushed by TV ads and how you can combat them with the simple facts.

What we've looked at up to now is misinformation about food. Another basic cause of poor eating habits is the misuse of food.

The Misuse of Food

From an objective standpoint, food is just that material we consume in order to keep us going. Human beings, however, are not very objective, and food has taken on a lot of other associations. In some ways this is fine—for example, we can enjoy a meal as a social occasion, as a time when we share something that provides pleasure. Food can also be misused. This is particularly true of parents who, after all, pretty much control what and when children eat. Here are some of the common ways in which food is misused.

Food as an indicator of affluence:

People who have gone short of food at some time in their lives sometimes become mildly obsessed with food. To reassure themselves that those days of poverty will never return, they keep the kitchen overstocked, eat more than necessary, and insist that their children do the same. The child who protests that he has had enough is likely to receive a lecture on the bad old days and on the children of India who would supposedly give their right arms for that spare rib. Eventually it becomes easier to stuff yourself than to listen to that. The further we get away from the time of the Depression, the less common this attitude is. However, some people who have never gone hungry consider the quantity as well as the quality of their food as a reflection of their success.

Food as a reward:

"Do your chores and you can have an extra dessert."

"Behave yourself and Daddy will buy you a candy bar."

"Get ready for bed now and Mommy will bring you in a snack."

These are all typical ways in which parents use food as a reward. The withholding of food likewise is frequently used as a punishment. The problem with this is that children soon get the impression that what sort of food one eats and when one eats depends upon whether one has been a good boy or girl. They really should be learning that good boys and girls have the same nutritional needs as bad boys and girls. We recognize the value of rewards in shaping kids' behavior (in fact that's an important part of our approach to changing eating habits), but the point is that food is not a good reward to use. In Chapter Seven, you'll find out about rewards that are effective and appropriate.

Food as a consolation:

Children encounter lots of disappointments: an exam failure, a ball game lost, a date turned down. For want of a better response, some mothers say something like, "Never mind. Here, have some cake." Food, usually sweet food, is offered as one of life's consolation prizes. This easily becomes part of a vicious circle. The fat child will encounter more social disappointments than the slim child. If he or she turns to food for consolation, that leads to further weight gain, which leads to further problems and on and on.

Food as a diversion:

Bored children are a pain in the neck. The busy parent has only so much time and so much patience. Sooner or later, parents fall back on suggestions like "go outside and play," or "sit down and watch television," or "go and fix yourself a little snack." Alas, the last two are more common and often appear in combination. When this becomes a habit, it's very difficult to change. The child will head for the kitchen every time he or she is bored or needs a break and can't think of anything better to do than to throw together a nice peanut butter and jelly sandwich.

In all these ways, food assumes psychological values. The legitimate role of food is as a source of nutrition and as an enjoyable experience for the taste buds. During the next few days, analyze your own behavior and that of your spouse and children to see whether you tend to use food as a reward, a consolation, or a remedy for boredom. If so, the sooner you stop and restore food to its proper role, the easier it will be for your child to slim down.

Chapter Summary

In all likelihood your child's weight problem is not due to glandular problems, heredity, or a phase of growing up. A physical examination will probably confirm that your child is overweight for two reasons: too much and the wrong kinds of food and too little exercise.

There are several reasons why children don't eat sensibly. Television is a powerful source of misinformation, and it pressures parents and children to buy and eat junk food. Parents also must stop misusing food as a reward, as a consolation prize, as a diversion, or to show they've "made it." When food is restored to its rightful place as a source of nutrition and a treat for the taste buds, it becomes easy for children to develop good eating habits.

3

What to Eat

Is Your Child Suffering from Malnutrition?

Say the word "malnutrition" and people automatically think of a skinny child in India or Africa. What if we tell you that malnutrition is a serious problem in the United States; do you assume that's only true in Appalachia? If so, you're wrong. Malnutrition is a problem not only in the ghettoes and the poor rural areas. Often it's a serious problem in the middle-class neighborhoods all over this country.

Malnutrition simply means "imperfect or faulty nutrition." It means that people aren't getting the nourishment they need from the food they eat. It's possible to eat a lot, in fact to be overweight and still have malnutition because you're not eating the right kind of foods. In extreme forms this leads to a variety of diseases. More typically it leads to a lack of energy, a poor complexion, and weight problems. Years ago malnutrition occurred in this country because people didn't have enough money. If they couldn't afford meat and cheese and eggs, they didn't get enough protein. If they couldn't afford fresh fruit and vegetables, they didn't get enough vitamin C. Fortunately, there are inexpensive sources of protein (like beans and peanut butter), and it's not costly to grow your own vegetables if you have access to a small plot of land. Nowadays our problem is the opposite: We have too much money (read on before you deny it). We value time more than money; so instead of cooking meals from fresh ingredients, we buy "convenience foods" that have lost much of their nutritive value and are stuffed with preservatives and dyes. We are in a hurry to get to the movies or the bowling alley or the color TV, so we eat at "fast food" places and sacrifice variety for the sake of convenience. And we no longer like to make a formal occasion out of mealtimes; so we combine hurried, skimpy meals with lots of filling snacks.

It would be unfair to suggest that all this has happened because we don't care about ourselves and our families. Like it or not, the pace of life has increased. Cooking and eating are subject to the same pressures as are other activities. More and more women are finding they want or need to work and are less willing or able to spend time slaving in the kitchen. Not all that many men want to take on part of the job—it's so much easier to go to the McDonald's or buy half a chicken from the Colonel or shove a TV dinner into the oven for 20 minutes.

It's not possible to turn back the clock even if we wanted to do so. However, even given the pressures of modern life, it's possible—and not too difficult—to come up with a menu that is nutritionally correct and at the same time enjoyable. Of course this is especially important for children, who need nutrients not only for their day-to-day activities but also for growth.

Before we describe a balanced diet and the nutrients it provides, let's take a closer look at the enemy: junk foods and especially sugar.

Why All the Fuss About Sugar?

There's a lot of money to be made in selling junk food. We mean the sugar-coated, puffed-up goodies that sell for a dime or quarter for an ounce or two. We mean the candy bars that get gloppier all the time. We mean the chemical milk shakes that have only a very distant relationship to ice cream. In other words, we mean the foods your child probably likes the most. Your children are taught to crave these products because they are pitched on television with a frequency of repetition that makes the Chinese Water Torture look mild by comparison.

Why should advertisers spend so much time and money selling Sugar Whackies and Caramel Crumbos instead of pushing healthful foods like plain yogurt or carrots? If you said "profit," go to the head of the class. High carbohydrate foods are cheap to make. If you puff them full of air, coat them with chocolate, encrust them with sugar, and put them in a fancy wrapper, you can sell them at an outrageous price. Protein foods don't serve the profit motive; for the most part they're too expensive to begin with. Vegetables don't either; what can you do to a carrot that will justify charging ten or twenty times what it cost you? We're talking about big money—the cereals alone are a $900 million a year business.

A lot of junk foods are made largely of sugar. So what's

wrong with sugar? The fact is that sugar is full of "empty" calories. That is, it provides calories but no nutritional value: no protein, no vitamins, no minerals. If you let a child fill up on sugary foods, you then have to cram him or her full of all sorts of other foods on top of that to make sure he or she is getting the nutrition required. Additionally, sugary foods not only contribute to tooth decay, but some, ice cream for instance, also contain fats as well.

Many people are under the impression that sugar is good for an instant shot of energy. But the best source of energy is a balanced diet. A good comparison is between the worker who eats a substantial, varied breakfast and the worker who has a sweet cup of coffee and a sugar-coated doughnut. The complete breakfast is steadily converted into energy all morning long. The dose of sugar merely raises the level of glucose in the blood sharply for a short time. Then the sugar addict is likely to go back to feeling listless until he can get his hands on a candy bar for another quick fix.

We can't expect young children to know all this, but isn't it amazing that more adults aren't aware of these facts? Not really. A tremendous amount of money goes into glossing them over. So we end up with a television commercial in which a once-famous actress tells us that although it's tempting to cut back on food these days, she'd never skimp on her children. She buys them "wholesome" Hostess Ho Ho's, Twinkies, and Cupcakes. Certainly the homemaker who does have to cut back would do well to eliminate such concoctions from her children's diet.

Another example is a full-page ad in a general circulation magazine. The color photo features a hand holding a candy bar with a bite missing. The inside of the bar is some sort of white cream, the outside a caramel covering with chunks of nuts stuck in it. In the background, somewhat out of focus, is a beaming boy with a covetous look in his eyes. Here's the text:

Kids, sugar, and psychology

Do you have that little impulse to say "no no" whenever you see your little one enjoying something with sugar in it? Lots of mothers have this prejudice. But, in fact, sugar can often do kids quite a bit of good. Sugar puts in the energy kids need in a form kids like. It not only helps youngsters stoke up fast, but the good natural sweetness gives them a sense of satisfaction and well-being. Nutritionists say that sugar, as an important carbohydrate, has a place in a balanced diet. A diet that includes the right kinds and right amounts of protein, vitamins, minerals, and fats, as well as carbohydrates. Sugar. It isn't just good flavor; it's good food.

To which we might add, it's even better business. Of course sugar "has a place in a balanced diet." But it's a much smaller place than it currently occupies in most people's diets. And that sense of "satisfaction and well-being" that kids get from sugar is likely to make them say they're full when you offer them food that *is* nutritious. No matter what the ads say, sugar is *not* good food.

Here's another example of how advertising can mislead the adult consumer. This one comes from Great Britain, in the form of a large newspaper ad. The picture is of half a dozen runners whooshing by so fast that they are just a blur. The headline: "Sheer energy, from Mr. Cube." Mr. Cube is a cute cartoon character who symbolizes Tate & Lyle Sugar. This is the text of the ad:

For sporting success, you need a balanced diet—and loads of energy. As everyone does, every day of their lives. And one of the cheapest ways of getting the energy you need is with Tate & Lyle's pure, British refined sugar. Just look at the energy-per-penny table and you'll see what we mean.

Incidentally, Redpath Sugars Limited, Tate & Lyle's subsidiary in Canada, is official supplier of sugar to the 1976 Olympic Games.

The "energy-per-penny table" reveals that granulated sugar gives 157 calories per penny while cheese gives a mere 39 calories per penny and roast sirloin of beef a pitiful 16 calories per penny. It's not surprising that the housewife with a shrinking food budget might assume from this that the best use of her money would be to cut back on cheese and meat and serve lots of sugar-saturated foods. That is the exact opposite of what she should do. A diet has more to it than simply loading up with as many calories as possible. Cheese and meat, both high in protein, are far superior to granulated sugar. If you looked at the diets of athletes, you'd find they're heavy on protein. Athletes go out of their way to consume sugar only when engaging in extremely demanding exercise in which a very temporary boost is needed.

If your child needs a pick-me-up between meals, he or she can get it from a piece of fresh fruit. Fruit sugar provides quick energy but not the drastic rush caused by refined, granulated cane sugar. Fruit sugar is also not as devastating to your child's teeth.

In several of the advertisements we've discussed, the advertisers suggested that candy or pastries are "wholesome." When a food is said to be wholesome, it presumably contains large amounts of vitamins, minerals, carbohydrates, and protein. Advertisers like the word because it sounds good but isn't very specific. It doesn't tell you how much of any nutrient there is, and it down-plays the presence of sugar and chemical preservatives.

Freshly baked pastries at your local bakery at least lack the chemical preservatives required for the "shelf life" of commercial brands. If there is anything wholesome about these candy and pastry products, it is whatever is included over and above the sugar, artificial flavoring, and the long list of added chemicals. Typically, the "wholesome" refers to the cornstarch and sometimes to eggs and milk. These incredients can be obtained directly, without the additional harmful ingredients.

The following chart shows the nutrients in cupcake mix made with eggs, milk, and chocolate icing, compared with the nutrients in eggs alone and skim milk alone. You can see that most of the protein in the cupcakes comes from the eggs, iron from eggs, potassium from eggs, vitamin A from eggs, thiamine from eggs and milk, and riboflavin from eggs and milk. If your child ate the same amounts of egg instead of cupcakes, he or she would consume less than half the calories and well over twice the protein.

The chart also compares the "wholesomeness" of chocolate-flavored caramel roll with that of Swiss pasteurized process cheese. An equal amount of cheese, while yielding fewer calories, provides twelve times the amount of protein.

Sugar and Tooth Decay

It is well known that ordinary table sugar is one of the main causes of tooth decay. Bacteria normally found in the mouth ferment the sugar. Fermented sugar forms an acid strong enough to dissolve tooth enamel. The worst form of sugar is that found in candies, especially caramels, which stick to the teeth over long periods of time. Refined sugar in any product, even breakfast cereal, is deadly to teeth. A study of 500 five year olds revealed that the children experienced a caries (tooth decay) increase which had a linear relation to the number of between-meal snacks they ate. Specifically, those who had one snack had a caries score of 4.8; those who had two snacks had a score of 5.7; three snacks, 8.5; and four or more snacks, 9.8. The research concluded that more important than how much sugar is eaten is how *often* sugar is eaten. In other words, frequent sugary snacks throughout the day do more dental damage than one meal containing lots of sugar.

Lest you think we're on some personal antisugar campaign, let us quote a statement issued by a White House conference on children and health:

Candies, confections, and beverages containing sucrose (refined sugar) should not be ingested by children between meals. Food manufacturers should limit sucrose in foods primarily intended for consumption by children. Education of the consumer on this point is essential.

As an intelligent consumer you will have to be careful

	Food Energy Calories	Protein Grams	Carbohydrate Grams	Calcium Milligrams	Phosphorus Milligrams
One pound of:					
Cupcake mix made with eggs, milk and chocolate icing	1,624	20.4	268.5	590	894
Eggs	739	58.5	4.1	245	930
Skim Milk	163	16.3	23.1	549	431
Chocolate-flavored caramel roll	4,796	10.0	375.1	308	540
Swiss pasteurized process cheese	1,610	119.8	7.3	4,023	3,933

to withstand not only the advertising that misinforms you as to the qualities of snack foods, but also the advertising that encourages you to misuse food. One television ad with which you may be familiar shows a family at a wedding. The child is fidgety and won't calm down until his mother gives him a LifeSaver. Thereafter the child is quiet, the wedding goes on, and presumably everyone lives happily ever after.

Iron Milligrams	Sodium Milligrams	Potassium Milligrams	Vitamin A International units	Thiamine Milligrams	Riboflavin Milligrams	Niacin Milligrams	Ascorbic Acid Milligrams
3.6	1,520	531	770	.16	.49	1.0	trace
10.4	553	585	5,350	.48	1.35	.3	0
.2	236	658	20	.16	.80	.3	5
8.2	894	558	trace	.07	.30	.6	trace
4.1	5,294	454	4,990	.03	1.81	.2	0

The advertisement tries to make you think the candy has successfully rewarded the child for sitting still and keeping quiet. What is really happening, though, is that the child is fidgety until his parent gives him candy. Then he rewards the parent by calming down. In order to get more candy, he has to become bothersome again. Then he does get more candy, and on it goes. The child is training his parent to give him more and more candy!

You will see in Chapter Six that there are effective ways to use rewards to guide your child into desirable behavior patterns (and you'll see it's done by rewarding good behavior, not bad behavior). But in any event, because the nutritional value of candy is so low compared to its drawbacks, you mustn't let yourself be conned into using it as a reward.

The Alternative: A Balanced Diet

Different kinds of food contain different combinations of nutrients. The best way to ensure that your child gets all the nutrients he or she needs is to give him or her a variety of food. There's nothing wrong with a meal consisting of a hamburger and french fries—unless your child gets into the habit of eating mostly hamburgers and french fries. The danger is that children will get into the habit of eating a very limited number of foods, and often these tend to be ones high in calories, too.

The following chart lists the nutrient groups, what they do for you, and which foods contain them. You may wonder why a child must get all of these nutrients. A lot of things may go wrong if he or she doesn't. The child may become listless, look pale and haggard, develop colds and other infections easily, and generally not feel well. Nutritionally balanced meals pay off in a healthy, energetic child who looks good and feels well.

At first glance it may seem a horrendous task to select a large enough variety of foods to supply all the essential nutrients. On closer examination, though, you'll see that many foods are repeated over and over in the list of nutrient sources. Some of the repeaters are milk, organ meats, fish, vegetables, fruit, and whole grains.

To sum it up, the key to adequate nutrition is to select foods from food groups that are a good source of many nutrients. Four basic food groups have been identified.

1) Milk and milk products such as cheese, yogurt, and buttermilk.
2) Meat and eggs, especially organ meats such as liver, heart, kidneys, and brain.
3) Vegetables and fruit, including green leafy vegetables.
4) Whole grain bread and cereals.

Nutrient groups	What they do for you	Which foods have them
Carbohydrates	Provide energy	Grains, vegetables
Fats	Provide energy; carry fat soluble vitamins	Organ meats, vegetable oils
Proteins	Essential for growth; regulating water balance; forming hormones, enzymes, antibodies; warding off infections	Milk, meat, whole grains, fish, eggs
Water	Essential for digestion, circulation, regulating body temperature, etc.	

Nutrient groups	What they do for you	Which foods have them
Vitamins: fat soluble		
A, D, E, K	Essential for eyesight, good complexion, healthy hair, several regulating functions, healing and protection from infection	Liver, milk, eggs, green leafy vegetables, whole grain, organ meats
Vitamins: water soluble		
B complex, B_1, B_2, B_6, B_{12}, biotin, folic acid, niacin, pantothenic acid, C	Essential for healthy skin and joints, resisting disease, metabolism, formation of red blood cells	Whole grains, green leafy vegetables, eggs, fruits, organ meats, milk, fish
Macrominerals:		
Calcium, phosphorus, magnesium, potassium, sodium, chlorine, sulphur	Essential in forming bones and other tissue, regulating body functions	Milk, meat, fruit, green leafy vegetables, whole grains, nuts
Trace Minerals:		
Iron, copper, iodine, fluorine, cobalt, manganese, zinc	Essential in forming hemoglobin in the blood, for hair and skin coloring, hormone production, strengthening teeth	Dark green leafy vegetables, egg yolks, shellfish, nuts, raisins, tea, bran

There is no one "miracle" diet. As you plan your meals, ask yourself these questions:

Am I serving a variety of meats, not just beef and chicken?

Am I serving salads at least three times a week?

Is there fresh fruit around the house?

Am I serving a cereal that doesn't have too much sugar (for example, shredded wheat)?

Do I serve milk or fruit juice or water with meals instead of soda pop?

Do I serve a variety of vegetables, perhaps in soups as well as with the main course?

Once you are able to answer "yes" to these questions, your child will be well on the way to having a balanced diet. The other question is *how much* food to serve your child. That depends upon your child's energy needs.

Estimating Your Child's Energy Needs

Your child needs food for energy. He or she uses energy in several ways:

Your child requires energy to perform all of the automatic functions like the pumping of the heart, breathing, and the digestion of food. These functions use up energy whether your child is thinking about them or not. The amount of energy required for the automatic functions is called "basal metabolism."

The second purpose for which energy is needed is to move the body or parts of it. Every movement made, even just lifting a finger, consumes energy. Of course the more weight that is moved, the faster it's moved, and the farther it's moved, the more energy is required.

The third use of energy is for growth. Infants may use as many as one calorie out of seven just for this purpose.

Energy needs vary, even among children of the same age. The factors that make a difference are the child's activity level, whether he or she is in a growth spurt, and the child's weight. The most rapid growth occurs during the infant's first year and again during adolescence, so these are two times when lots of energy is needed. As a general guideline, the Food and Nutrition Board recommends the following calorie levels for children:

	Number of Calories
Children:	
1–3	1300
3–6	1600
6–9	2100
Boys:	
9–12	2400
12–15	3000
15–18	3400
Girls:	
9–12	2200
12–15	2500
15–18	2300

Controlling Calories

It isn't necessary to become fanatical about counting how many calories your child consumes; this would make your life and your child's life miserable. But you should familiarize yourself with the caloric value of the basic foods and make sure you're not serving mainly high-calorie meals. Appendix A gives the caloric value of most of the foods you're likely to serve, and with it you'll be able to find low-calorie substitutes for some of the excessively rich foods you may now be serving too often. If you provide moderate-size portions of a variety of foods and eliminate snacks, you will automatically be reducing your child's calorie intake. In Chapter Five we will ask you to count calories for just one week. When you are done, look back to the chart of recommended calorie consumption. If your tally is considerably higher than the recommended number, you'll know you have to cut down on how much your child eats or cut down on the high-calorie foods in his or her diet.

Chapter Summary

The overweight child usually eats too much of the wrong kind of food. Worst of all are sugar-laden cereals, candies, and other junk food. These foods fill up your child and make him or her less receptive to eating nutritional foods. They also rot your child's teeth. They are heavily and cleverly advertised to convince children that

candy is wholesome, desirable, almost essential. Cutting
down and eventually eliminating such foods from your
child's diet is the single most important thing you can do
to ensure that he or she slims down and is healthy. The
key to good nutrition is serving a balanced diet. If the
meals you serve contain representatives of the four basic
food groups, your child will get all of the required nutrients. Although you need not continually count calories,
you can estimate your child's energy needs and from time
to time compare this to actual intake and adjust your
menus accordingly.

4

What Exercise Has to Do With It

The last chapter was concerned with what your child puts into the body. This chapter deals with what your child does with that body. People often naively assume that children automatically get the necessary amount of exercise. They suppose that even if they appear to be sluggish at home they must be actively participating in physical education courses at school. This assumption overestimates the job P.E. courses do and underestimates the ingenuity a child can use to get out of an activity he doesn't enjoy. One of the authors (Wolff) can personally attest to this fact, having spent most of his childhood in right field.

The most common form of exercise indulged in by kids is that of competitive games: baseball, football, volley ball, basketball, and so forth. The reason that the overweight child doesn't enjoy these games is quite simple: He or she is usually not very good at them. The extra pounds reduce speed, agility, and endurance. The fat kid is picked last when sides are being chosen, and this kind of rejection adds insult to injury.

At the junior and senior high school level, another psychological factor is involved. At these levels students shower after their physical education classes, and there is no way to hide flabbiness in the shower. Already sensitive young people may dread this ultimate exposure of their condition and hate P.E. all the more. For many it is a spur to think of ways of getting out of physical education classes altogether.

These factors are the elements of a vicious circle: The child's overeating makes him or her fat and unlikely to participate in games and other forms of exercise; in turn, the lack of exercise doesn't give the child the chance to burn off calories and therefore adds to the weight problem.

There is, of course, a health danger associated with inactivity. Our bodies are designed to be used, and they gain strength from use. Muscles that are exercised increase in size and strength. Muscles that aren't used become weak and lose their tone. Similarly, the heart and lungs benefit by having their capacity stretched. When periodically called upon to do more than is usually required (such as when running), the body is ready to do more in an emergency (such as when it is under attack by a disease). Heart attacks and disease associated with being out of shape don't usually strike children, but the out-of-shape adult formed poor exercise habits in childhood and certainly the healthy child is more likely to be a healthy adult. Having gotten into the habit of enjoying exercise, he or she will be more willing to continue that exercise in later life. Therefore it should be clear that exercise is desirable for *all* people, not just the overweight. For the overweight, it has the added advantage of leading to weight loss.

There is another, lesser known way that exercise helps

some people to slim down. There is a control center in your brain that tells you how much food you should be eating. When you need more, it signals that you are hungry. For people of normal weight, this control center works correctly. For people who are overweight, it *may* still be working correctly, but these people eat even when they do not feel hungry—perhaps to enjoy the taste of a particular food, or because they think it would be rude to turn down a second helping, or because they have gotten used to misusing food in one of the ways mentioned in Chapter Two. These people have to learn to pay attention to the control center and eat only when it's sending out hunger signals as well as learning to eat the right kinds of foods. But there are other people whose control centers are, in effect, out of control. They keep getting hunger signals even if they've just finished a full meal. Experiments have shown that these people are the ones who get almost no exercise. Their control centers resume working properly some time after these people have increased the amount of exercise they get. If you have a child who constantly whines, "I'm hungry," one possibility is that this is simply his or her way of getting attention from you. But it is also possible that the child genuinely feels hungry and that an increase in exercise will actually *decrease* his or her appetite.

Every movement, every activity burns up calories, including just sitting around or sleeping. Even if you're not moving, you need to keep your heart and lungs and other organs working. The more vigorous the activity, the more calories consumed. Since calorie reduction is the only practical and effective means of losing weight, we recommend a two-pronged attack: Reduce the number of calories your child takes in, and increase the number of calories your child burns up. A little of each of these measures is an easy-to-take and effective combination.

By the way, parents sometimes say that someone else's child can eat like a pig without gaining any weight while their poor child seems to put on pounds no matter what. No healthy person can eat beyond his or her requirements without gaining weight. The other child may have a slightly different metabolic rate, but more importantly, he or she is probably getting a lot more exercise. One study of teenage girls showed that a group of overweight girls actually consumed *fewer* calories than a group of girls of normal weight. The latter got a lot more exercise, and that's what made the difference.

To see the calorie consumption of various kinds of activities, check the Approximate Calorie Consumption chart. The specific number of calories used up depends upon your child's weight and metabolism, but these approximate figures for adults will give you the idea and allow you to compare various kinds of exercise. You may be a bit discouraged by the fact that it takes 16 minutes of cycling to work off the effects of eating an ounce of caramels, or 40 minutes of swimming to use up the calories contained in 3 ounces of hard candy. But remember the health payoffs of exercise, and use this as a reminder not to let your child get his or her hands on caramels or hard candy too often.

Helping Your Child Get More Exercise

What can a parent do to encourage a child to get more exercise? It isn't necessary to convert the guest room into a gym or to build a sauna in the garage. We advocate a gradual, nonpunishing increase, which will go hand-in-hand with your reform of your child's diet.

You can begin by having a talk with your child's physical education teacher, especially if your boy or girl is still in elementary school. Find out to what extent the P.E. course incorporates individual exercise (such as calisthenics) as opposed to team sports in which the poor performer easily gets lost. Ask whether your child tends to hang back or seems to be experiencing difficulties. Explain to the teacher that you are working on a program to lower your child's weight and that you would appreciate his or her aid. The teacher can encourage your child to take a more active part and praise the child when he or she does well. Some teachers organize competitive games into teams of comparable ability so that each child has the opportunity to experience success.

Physical education teachers are so used to dealing only with the parents of the stars (for example, the kids on the after-school teams), that they will be pleasantly surprised to be approached by a parent who recognizes the importance of exercise for average or below-average performers. A sure way to enlist the continuing cooperation of the instructor is to send a thank-you note (which also serves as a reminder) after a couple of months. If the teacher was cooperative, a note to that effect to the principal is also a good idea.

There are also a number of things you can do to ensure that your children get more exercise in the hours outside of school. Here are a few of the most effective and least burdensome exercises:

APPROXIMATE CALORIE CONSUMPTION
OF VARIOUS EXERCISES

1. Archery .... 5.2   Calories per minute

2. Canoeing .... 3.0   "
   (2.5 mph)

3. Canoeing .... 7.0   "
   (4.0 mph)

4. Climbing .... 10.7   "
   (light load & slope)

5. Climbing .... 13.2   "
   (heavy load & slope)

6. Cross-country
   running .... 10.6   "

7. Cycling .... 4.5   "
   (5.5 mph)

8. Cycling .... 7.0   "
   (9.4 mph)

9. Dancing:
   Slow .... 5.7   "
   Medium 7.0
   Fast 10.0

10. Football .... 8.9   "

11. Gardening:
    Digging .... 8.6   "
    Weeding 5.0

12. Horseback riding:
    Walking .... 3.0   "
    Trotting 8.0

13. Scrubbing and
    kneeling .... 3.4   "

14. Skiing:
    Hard snow,
    3.7 mph .... 9.9   "
    Max. speed 18.6

15. Swimming .... 8.0   "

16. Tennis .... 7.0   "

17. Walking:
    2 mph .... 2.6   "
    3.5 mph 3.6

Walking

This is one of the best all-round, nonstrenuous exercises because it helps the heart, lungs, and legs to gain strength. As you can see from the chart, it uses up about 3.6 calories a minute. Until your child is old enough to have a car, you're in a position to control his or her transportation. If your boy or girl has a bike, here's a good rule of thumb: Have your child walk to the destinations to which he or she usually cycled and have your child cycle to the places to which you previously drove him or her. Obviously sometimes there are safety considerations that prevent this, but particularly if your children are ten or older, are you sure that you really need to drive them to school any more? Couldn't they walk or pedal there without undue hardship? Similarly, if you need something from a nearby store, couldn't your child walk or bike there for you?

If you are alert to the possibilities, you'll think of a lot of occasions on which your child could increase the amount of walking he or she does. Incidentally, one way to get your child into the walking habit is to make a walk around the neighborhood a family affair, maybe right after dinner. It'll help the digestion, tune you all in to what's happening around you, and give you the chance to be closer as a family. Besides—admit it—you're getting a little flabby yourself, and a walk won't hurt you either.

Bicycling

The last few years have seen an impressive upswing in the popularity of cycling. Bicycle sales are up, and cities and towns are establishing bicycle lanes and paths that make this a much safer and more convenient mode of transportation than it used to be. Cycling is an excellent exercise. Like walking, it is a balanced exercise, by which we mean that it lets you exercise several parts of your body. It's also a practical way for kids to get around. If you haven't bought your boy or girl a bike, you may want to consider it. There's no need to splurge on a Mark 4000 Ten-Speed—a three-speed or even a one-speed will do the job —and a secondhand bike is fine if you'd like to save money. Most police departments have periodic auctions at which they dispose of unclaimed, recovered bicycles, and this is a good way to find a bargain.

If your child has a bike but has lost interest in it, it may be relatively easy to revive that interest: Repaint the bike (how about fluorescent orange?), or add streamers to it, hook up a speedometer. Any of these may be enough to send your child all over the neighborhood to show off the "new" bike. Bicycling is also a good family activity. It doesn't cost much to outfit Mom and Dad with a couple of secondhand bikes, setting the stage for nightly cycle tours or weekend bike trips.

Swimming

Even if you're not in a position to build a pool in your back yard, you probably don't live too far from a YMCA, YWCA, or community recreation center pool your child could use. If he or she is self-conscious, enroll your child in a beginner's swimming class: Everyone is too busy trying not to drown to notice who's fat and who's skinny. It also will give your child a useful skill for later life and an activity in which he or she can succeed. If your child does know how to swim, this is a factor you might want to take into account when planning the family vacation. If possible, structure it so that it gives your children (and you) lots of opportunities to get exercise.

Gardening and Other Chores

Many parents feel that giving their children chores to do helps kids develop a sense of responsibility. If the chores are carefully chosen, they can also help kids to get useful exercise. Gardening is required in most households, and weeding, mowing the lawn, and trimming the hedges are not too difficult for kids to handle. Previously mentioned were chores which involve walking and cycling, such as going on shopping errands. Chores are easily built into an incentives program, as explained in Chapter Seven.

Sports

We suggest you encourage your child to develop an interest in nonteam sports. These sports allow your child to play with others at his or her own level of ability and they are easier to carry on into adulthood. They include tennis, badminton, bowling, archery, golf, water-skiing, and snow-skiing. These sports vary in difficulty and in the degree of competitiveness they entail. But if you take your cue from your geographical location and from your knowledge of your kids, you may be able to help them get started on an activity that will serve them well for the rest of their lives. Once again, some of these sports are suitable for family participation. Starting out to learn tennis or another sport from (or with) an accepting parent may be less threatening to self-conscious children than being immersed in a class with other children.

The best thing is to indicate that you would support this kind of activity (for example, by picking up the tab for a series of lessons) and let the children make the decision for themselves. It may take them a while to revise their own self-image enough to see themselves as being potentially active in sports.

Exercise Programs

Most of the exercises we have suggested are less demanding than a specific exercise program that includes push-ups, sit-ups, and so forth. For this reason they will also be more acceptable to overweight kids. But if your child becomes actively interested in improving his or her physical condition, we suggest you get a copy of a book entitled *Aerobics*, by Dr. Kenneth Cooper.

Dr. Cooper has devised an exercise program to be done in the home. It provides a good variety of exercises, and it's set up so it progressively increases in difficulty. This last point is especially important for the overweight child, who is used to failure and must be shown that he or she can succeed at one level and move on. With this program, kids experience success from the moment they start, moving gradually to the goal level for their age.

From among the approaches we have presented in this chapter, you will be able to design a way to increase the exercise your boy or girl is getting. That is one of the ten most important weight-related behaviors with which you can help your child. All ten are further discussed in the next chapter.

Chapter Summary

Overweight children usually are less physically active than children of average weight. Because their bulk slows them down, overweight kids aren't as good in competitive sports, and this tends to turn them off to all kinds of exercise. A good exercise program will help the slimming process and have health payoffs. Parents should gain the cooperation of the physical education teacher as well as encouraging their children to exercise during nonschool hours. Useful forms of exercise include walking, bicycling, swimming, gardening, and a variety of nonteam sports. For a more formal exercise program we recommend Dr. Kenneth Cooper's *Aerobics*.

5

The Ten Most Important Eating Behaviors

In this chapter, we take a closer look at ten kinds of behavior related to eating and to weight control. In our experience these ten behaviors hold the key to losing weight and developing an adequate, sensible diet. After you have read about each one, we will invite you to assess your child's current performance of that behavior. The information you jot down now will be crucial when you get to Chapter Eight and design a weight-loss program for your child; so do take the time. Also don't be discouraged if your child has problems with most of these ten behaviors. In the next two chapters, you'll find out how to use psychology and incentives to change these behaviors one at a time.

1. Eating a Good Breakfast

Many children are used to seeing Dad or Mom rush off in the morning having had only a doughnut and a cup of coffee. For some strange reason, people are almost proud to say, "Oh, I never eat breakfast." Maybe it's supposed to show us how busy (and therefore important) they are, or to demonstrate how much willpower they have. It's a habit picked up easily by children as well, and it's a foolish one. In many ways, breakfast is the most important meal of the day. It makes sense to provide your body with fuel when it is most likely to need it, and for students and workers alike the morning is a time of heavy demands. It's the time you set your pace for the whole day; a sluggish morning, or one in which you're distracted by the rumblings in your stomach is a bad way to start. And the people who say, "I don't need anything in the mornings," are the ones lining up at the candy machine during the first coffee break or recess.

Some people claim to have a revulsion to food in the morning. It's true that it can be tough to look a soft-boiled egg in the eye at 6:00 A.M., particularly if alcohol figured in the events of the previous evening. But breakfast doesn't have to consist of a soft-boiled egg, and it doesn't have to be so huge that forcing it down is a revolting prospect. If you and your family are used to eating nothing for breakfast, start by serving each person a glass of orange juice and a piece of toast. When they're used to that, add a small portion of cereal. In this way you can very gradually train your digestive systems and your psyches to get used to the idea of having a nutritious meal early in the day.

The coffee-and-a-doughnut people recognize they need something, but they're getting the wrong things. With the coffee they're trying to jolt themselves awake with a shot of caffeine. With the doughnut they're trying to get a fix of quick energy by eating a sugary food. This works quickly, but it wears off just as quickly. Even before midmorning they're back to feeling weak, and perhaps they then have another quick shot by eating a candy bar or another doughnut. Since we've been comparing food to a fuel, we might say that eating this sort of breakfast is like fueling your car with a gasoline that makes it lurch forward a short distance and then die, as opposed to one that lets the car run smoothly for a long time.

The child's equivalent of coffee with doughnuts is a bowl of sweet cereal. These cereals are sold on the basis of their shape, their color, whether or not they snap or crackle, the prizes in the boxes, and the cartoon characters who advertise them on television. Some years ago the decision as to how much sugar to put on cereal was up to the consumer. As we've mentioned, now the great majority of cereals geared to the children's market are presweetened (this doesn't keep some kids from shoveling on extra sugar, of course). A couple of years ago these kinds of cereals were analyzed and it was discovered that children could actually get more nutritional value by eating the box the cereals came in than by eating the cereals themselves! After that publicity, the manufacturers added some cheap vitamins and proclaimed their cereals to be "New!" and "Vitamin fortified!" There *are* some sensible cereals on the market. Look at the contents tables of the cereals you're considering. When manufacturers list ingredients, they do so in order of quantity. So when sugar is listed as first or second, you know that particular cereal is full of sugar. The best strategy is to switch your children to an unsweetened cereal and to take charge of the sugar bowl. Gradually decrease the amount of sugar you spoon on until you are serving the cereal without any sugar at all. Cutting up fresh fruit into the cereal is a good way of making it a bit sweeter and more palatable to your children.

We have seen what constitutes a bad breakfast. What's

a good breakfast, then? Here are three sample menus that would be reasonable for a child:

A large glass of milk
Piece of toast (preferably made with wholewheat bread)
One or two eggs
Fruit

Small glass of fruit juice
Glass of milk
One or two sausages
Toast

Small glass of juice
Bowl of *unsweetened cereal* with half a banana cut up
    and added, with milk
Small glass of milk
Small piece of bread with cheese spread

There are lots of other foods that are good at breakfast: cold or warm ham, beans on toast, bacon, omelettes of various kinds, oatmeal, fruit salad, etc. To make breakfast interesting and to avoid a diet too high in cholesterol, it's best to add some variety rather than serving the traditional two eggs with bacon every morning.

One final point regarding breakfast. If you add some calories in the morning, you've got to subtract calories at some other point in the day. Part of this may occur naturally because your child will feel less of a craving for snacks between meals. But if your youngsters used to come to lunch in a ravenous state, you should now also be able to cut back a bit on that meal. The same goes for dinners.

The typical pattern in America is no breakfast, a moderate lunch, and a heavy dinner. The pattern should be turned around. It makes more sense for you and your family to have a moderate breakfast, a moderate lunch, and a light dinner. For the most part, the evening is the least demanding time of the day, spent on unstrenuous activities like watching television, doing homework, reading, going to the movies, or visiting friends. For these activities you don't need a huge infusion of calories. This doesn't mean you have to stop serving delicious evening meals, only that you can safely cut back a bit on their quantity and go easy on desserts.

Now take a minute to jot down on the next page the kind of breakfast your child usually eats, if any. You'll use this information a little later, in designing a weight-loss program for your child.

2. Controlling Snacks

You will have less difficulty controlling what your children eat at mealtimes than you will controlling what they eat between meals. However, the control of snacks is essential. Not only do they contain loads of empty calories, they also blunt your child's appetite so that he or she is less willing to eat the nutritious food you serve at mealtimes. There are several things you can do. First, don't buy junk food like candy bars, potato chips, candied popcorn, and gooey cupcakes. Children eat junk food for the same reason a mountain climber climbs a mountain: because it's there. Your kids' attention may be caught by the bright package, or the fact that a brother or sister is having a

MY CHILD'S TYPICAL BREAKFAST

snack, or by thinking if they fill up now they won't have to eat as much at dinner. TV ads also trigger snacking. If the snack food simply isn't there to be eaten, there's not much the kids can do about it.

Your eventual goal is cutting down drastically on between-meal eating, but as an interim measure you can provide some reasonably healthy snacks. A "sweet tooth" is something we acquire, not something with which we are born. We can lose it again. Once children get out of the candy habit they may actually feel repulsed by the sweet messes they used to crave. This takes a little while to happen, but knowing that it will happen should make your job easier. In the meantime, oranges, apples, bananas, grapes, and other kinds of fruit are attractive and tasty snacks. So are some vegetables; try keeping some carrot and celery sticks in a bowl of water in the refrigerator. If your child is used to ice cream, switch to jello or to yogurt (preferably natural yogurt by itself or with fresh fruit cut into it, rather than the preflavored kind, which contains sugar and preservatives).

Another important step you can take is switching your kids away from soda pop. Fruit juices are a good alternative, but be sure you are serving pure fruit juices, not "juice drinks." If you look at the labels of fruit drinks, you'll see these are mostly water with loads of sugar and a little flavoring and food coloring. Vitamin C is cheap, so some manufacturers add a bit of it and call this mixture a healthy drink. You'd do better with a glass of water and a vitamin C pill, but if your child eats a reasonable amount of fruit, he or she won't need the vitamin C pill either. If your child comes in hot and thirsty after playing, encourage him or her to drink a glass of water first to quench the thirst before going on to drink anything else.

Finally, if you are in the habit of giving your child a bedtime snack, gradually phase this out. Children, especially younger ones, like to feel secure before they go to sleep. Their call for a glass of milk and a snack before they can get to sleep is simply a bid for a little more attention, for a reassurance that Mommy or Daddy loves them. This is better done by spending more time with the kids at bedtime, maybe with a story or a brief talk about the events of the day or just a nice long hug—none of these are fattening, and they're more satisfying than an Oreo cookie.

So far we've talked about the eating your child does at home. It's harder keeping tabs on what happens outside of your house. Most likely, your child has two or three friends he or she visits. Sit down for a moment with the parents of these playmates and explain what you're doing. You don't have to try to convert them to good nutritional habits (although some of them probably will be interested in sharing what you've learned); just ask them not to serve a lot of snacks when your child is there. If there is one mother (maybe a chubby one) who doesn't want to get the message, have her son or daughter come to your house instead of letting your child go over there.

Even though they should know better many schools have candy machines. In many areas, Parent-Teacher Associations or even individual parents have succeeded in getting these machines removed, and you can give that a try. The schools get a share of the profits from these machines, so they may not want to ban them entirely; but perhaps they'll be willing to switch to machines that dispense fruit, crackers with cheese, yogurt, jello, and similar foods instead of candy bars.

If you have been giving your child lunch money and suspect it's going toward the candy machine instead of the school's hot meal, pack your child's lunch instead. It'll take a few minutes more of your time, but the results will be worth it.

Finally, it may help to control the flow of your child's allowance. If your child has his eye on a toy, offer to save the money for him (you can make up a "bankbook") until he's got enough. This discourages him from dribbling the money away on little things like candy bars.

We don't intend that you become a police officer or a spy, or that you absolutely forbid any snacks, but applying as many of these measures as seems sensible will help.

On the following page, write down the snacks that your child usually eats in the course of the day and also *when* he or she usually eats them. For example, it might be "peanut butter sandwich when he comes home from school," and "candy bar in the evening," and "milk and cookies just before bedtime." Again, you'll use this information later.

It will take only a few minutes to jot down those snacks eaten most often. You can do this from memory. In the next section you will find some charts for writing down the actual food your child eats each day for a week, including breakfasts and snacks. Those charts will help you to see that recording the actual food eaten each day gives you a different picture than the one you get by writing from memory. Both are important. Writing from memory gives you a list of the most frequently eaten snacks; but recording actual food eaten each day gives a moving

**SNACKS MY CHILD USUALLY EATS
AND THE TIMES THEY ARE EATEN**

picture which shows how one thing leads to another and what changes from day to day.

This may be a good place to congratulate you for filling out the charts provided so far in this book. If you have been writing down the points that were asked for, you have taken an important, positive step toward your goal. In a few weeks, after you have made changes in your child's eating pattern, you will be able to look back at these charts and see exactly how much the picture has improved.

3. Controlling Calories

Controlling calories is one half of the battle. The other half is making sure that the calories come in the form of a balanced diet. First, calories. We already know that your child is taking in more calories than he or she is using up. And you'll remember that the caloric value of food isn't directly related to the quantity of the food. In other words, you can eat a pound of one kind of food and not take in any more calories than you would by eating a couple of ounces of another kind. It is helpful to know which foods are high in calories, which are moderate, and which are low; and this is easier than you may think. It's not necessary to weigh every ounce of food and compute down to the last calorie. Once you have looked up the kinds of meals you usually serve, you'll start to get a feel for the caloric value of the different kinds of foods.

On the next few pages are charts in which you should write down the meals your child eats during one week, and the approximate caloric value of each part of the meal. (So that you don't have to buy a separate calorie book,

Appendix A of this book lists the most common foods and how many calories they contain.) Probably the easiest way to do this is to write down each day's food intake at the end of the day. Do this for a week. Use your best judgment in estimating how much of each kind of food your child has eaten. Be sure to ask about food eaten outside of the house and remember that liquids (other than water) are foods, too. You'll also have to take into account the ingredients of a dish. When writing down a spaghetti dinner, you'll have to break it down into the cheese, tomato paste, and meat, as well as the spaghetti. If you can't find the exact food you served, use the calorie figures of the food you think is most similar.

Complete these charts *before* you start adjusting your child's diet. If you've already made some changes as a result of what you've read so far, recreate a week's menu that's typical of what your child used to eat. Once again, you're gathering information that you'll use to decide what changes are required in your child's diet, so it is worth the few minutes of effort it takes.

4. Eating Balanced Meals

As you learned in the chapter on nutrition, it's essential that the food you serve provides your children with the right kinds of nutrients as well as a reasonable number of calories. Here is a review of the four basic food groups:

1) Milk and milk products such as cheese, yogurt, and buttermilk.

SUNDAY

Breakfast:

Lunch:

Dinner:

Snacks:

MONDAY

Breakfast:

Lunch:

Dinner:

Snacks:

TUESDAY

Breakfast:

Lunch:

Dinner:

Snacks:

WEDNESDAY

Breakfast:

Lunch:

Dinner:

Snacks:

THURSDAY

Breakfast:

Lunch:

Dinner:

Snacks:

FRIDAY

Breakfast:

Lunch:

Dinner:

Snacks:

SATURDAY

Breakfast:

Lunch:

Dinner:

Snacks:

2) Meat and eggs, especially organ meats such as liver, heart, kidneys, and brain.
3) Vegetables and fruit.
4) Whole grain bread and cereals.

A good rule of thumb is that the daily diet should include at least two portions of food from each of these groups. Remember to strive for variety in the diet. For example, rather than always filling the vegetable requirement with carrots and peas, experiment with lots of others. It will help to make mealtimes more interesting and prevent your children from becoming finicky eaters unwilling to try anything except the half-dozen dishes that they've had over and over. Equally important, it will help ensure that your children get a full range of vitamins and minerals.

In the previous section of this chapter you recorded all the food your child ate during the course of a week. Refer back to that now, and on the chart on the following pages write down the *number* of the food group for each food consumed each day. For example, if on a given day your child had a breakfast of a glass of milk, one fried egg, and a piece of toast, you'd write down 1, 2, and 4 (and another 1 if the toast was buttered). Do the same for the other meals and for snacks. This will let you examine whether your child has been eating a balanced diet on a day-to-day and weekly basis. If you find a lot of one kind of food and a shortage of another, you will see that some adjustment is required, and this will become part of your child's weight-loss program.

SUNDAY

Breakfast:

Lunch:

Dinner:

Snacks:

MONDAY

Breakfast:

Lunch:

Dinner:

Snacks:

TUESDAY

Breakfast:

Lunch:

Dinner:

Snacks:

WEDNESDAY

Breakfast:

Lunch:

Dinner:

Snacks:

THURSDAY

Breakfast:

Lunch:

Dinner:

Snacks:

FRIDAY

Breakfast:

Lunch:

Dinner:

Snacks:

SATURDAY

Breakfast:

Lunch:

Dinner:

Snacks:

5. Keeping Food in Its Place

In Chapter Two, we described some of the ways in which food can be misused:

as an indicator of affluence
as a reward
as a consolation
as a diversion

Since reading that chapter, perhaps you've had a chance to think about whether you have misused food in any of these ways or in other ways. If so, jot down examples on the next couple of pages. Please, be honest with yourself; no one other than you needs to look at the information you write in this book, and your honesty will benefit your boy or girl. Next to each of your examples, write down an alternate way you could handle the situation in the future. For example, having a chat with your child and telling him that you still love him and have confidence in him is much more a consolation than a double serving of a favorite snack. A new picture book or a jigsaw puzzle is a much

MISUSE OF FOOD   **ALTERNATIVES**

better remedy for boredom than plunking a kid down in front of a TV with a candy bar. The next chapter will give you many further examples of possible rewards.

Your attitudes and behavior in relation to food will serve as a model for your children, so it's helpful not to misuse food in relationship to yourself as well as in relationship to them. Give a little thought to other ways of rewarding, consoling, or diverting yourself as well. And finally, if you find your attitudes and knowledge about food is changing, pass some of this on to your children. You don't have to do it in a formal way; if your kids are watching you fix dinner, you can casually tell them a little about how the meat or vegetables you're cooking help to maintain and build up the body.

6. Getting Enough Exercise

Although it takes a lot of exercise to use up any significant number of calories, it has other benefits: It helps muscle tone, it improves general health, and it helps the self-image of the child who's gotten used to seeing himself or herself as a sluggish lump of flesh.

Chapter Four suggested a number of activities that could help your child get more exercise and suggested that you enlist the help of the physical education teacher. In Chapter Eight you'll decide which activities to encourage, but first you should have a clear picture of how much exercise your child gets now. On the following few pages, jot down the activities in which your child has engaged during the past week. Include anything beyond the minimum necessary to get out of bed, get dressed, eat, and walk out

EXERCISE SUMMARY

Monday:

Tuesday:

Wednesday:

Thursday:

EXERCISE SUMMARY

Friday:

Saturday:

Sunday:

the door. For example, each weekday might include a 10-minute walk to school, and one day might include a 15-minute bike ride. Without turning it into an inquisition you can ask your child about what he or she does during P.E. and in free time away from home. Again, it's not important that you be obsessive about this. The important thing is that you have a good general idea of how much exercise your child gets now, so that you'll be able to increase it gradually.

7. Easing Tension

There are two facts related to this behavior which may surprise you: Children as well as adults suffer from tension, and tension contributes to weight problems.

What we are talking about is muscle tension. Just like the fibers in a taut rope, when a muscle is tense its fibers are pulled up tight. They actually vibrate under the workload. A tense muscle burns up energy and builds up carbon dioxide and other waste materials. Eventually it becomes fatigued and begins to ache.

Muscles tense and then relax in physical activity such as walking up steps. Alternating between tension and rest keeps muscles in tone and working efficiently and contributes to good health. The continuous tension caused by stress does not benefit your health.

An example of tension caused by stress is the furrowed brow that sometimes results from worrying. If you're waiting for someone to come home to dinner and that person is late you start to worry: Did the car break down? Has there been an accident? Why hasn't he or she called? Tiny muscles pull the skin together between the eyebrows and the muscle tension continues until these muscles ache with fatigue. Finally they trigger a tension headache.

The normal stresses we encounter during a day cause a certain level of tension in various muscles. Common centers of muscle tension are the back of the neck, the throat, the abdomen, and across the shoulders.

Often tension caused by stress leads to overeating. Food that tastes good serves as a reward for having survived the stress. You usually relax while eating because the act of eating distracts you, and this relaxation soothes the muscles. For example, you may suffer a lot of stress getting the kids off to school in the morning, making sure they're properly dressed, have their books and homework and lunch money, and so forth. Once they're out the door you take a break by sitting down with your feet up and having a cup of coffee and a doughnut. Suddenly you feel much more relaxed, and you associate the relaxation with the food—it seems as though the food is *causing* the relaxation. Actually, what's allowing you to relax is the fact that the house no longer sounds like the barracks at the camp of Attila the Hun and the knowledge that now you can get down to doing what needs to be done for the rest of the day. If you allow yourself to believe that food is the answer to stress, you'll soon be in the habit of munching every time a problem crops up.

Tension also tends to make you irritable and to feel that nothing is going right. In this state of mind you're more likely to fall back on old, undesirable eating habits. You may even feel things are so bleak that it doesn't make any difference whether or not you lose weight.

Undoubtedly you can understand how stress leads to

tensions in adults, but perhaps you've never considered that the same thing happens to your children. Childhood problems may seem trifling from an adult viewpoint, but children see them from a child's viewpoint. Passing the spelling test is as important to a child as getting a promotion is to an adult. Having to get up to recite a poem in class is as worrying as making a business speech or addressing the P.T.A. And finally, imagine how you'd feel if you stepped into an elevator and a group of adults began to openly ridicule you because you're overweight. Why should your child feel any less distress when he or she is teased and called names by the other children? Your child may withdraw from the other kids at recess and head for the candy machine. When your child comes home and prepares a snack, a link is built up between food and relaxation, just as in our earlier example.

Relaxation is a skill, and it's easily acquired with a little practice. If your child shows signs of tension, have him or her sit down in a comfortable chair after coming home from school. Play soft music on the radio or stereo, and have your child relax each part of the body. You might say something like this:

Are you comfortable? Good. Don't think about anything, just listen to what I'm saying. We'll start with your left foot . . . let it relax . . . pretend it's made of stone, it's very heavy and it just lies there. Now do the same with your right foot . . . don't make it stiff, just pretend it's turning to stone all by itself . . . now the same thing is happening with your legs, all the way up to the knees . . .

You continue this process with the rest of the body and then ask your child to think of a pleasant, quiet scene for a few minutes, before getting up. If your child is older, you can get him or her to do this alone, once you've demonstrated the technique. If your child doesn't know what you mean by relaxing, compare it to how the child feels just before drifting off to sleep. You can also have the child make a fist, as hard as possible, and then let go; explain that the way the fist feels when it is let go is what you mean by relaxing.

If your child is tense, you'll discover that going through this relaxation exercise after school or just before dinner helps not only with overeating but may lead to a general improvement in behavior. If you're a bit tense as well, why not do this along with your child every day?

Use the following chart to decide whether tension is a problem for your child. Look for the tension cues listed and check the appropriate column. If you answer "Often" or "Sometimes" on two or more, relaxation is a skill your child should develop.

	Often	Sometimes	Never
1. Do the facial muscles appear tense? Is there tension around the eyes, forehead and/or mouth?			
2. Do the shoulders appear drawn up as if shrugging?			
3. Is the child fidgety as if trying to stimulate himself or herself?			

4. Is there tension in the
   voice? Is it higher
   pitched than usual?

8. Eating Slowly

When a plane is refueling, time means money to the airline. The more fuel that can be piped in quickly, the more pleased the passengers are, too, because they don't want to be held up any longer than necessary. What is appropriate at the airport isn't appropriate at the dinner table, but you'd never guess it from judging by the eating habits of some children. Especially for the overweight, eating can become a mechanical process instead of a pleasant as well as essential act. By cramming down food, children lose touch with its qualities and they lose touch with when to stop. Eating is part of the greater process of digesting the food and sorting and storing the nutrients. When eating is not done properly, the rest of the process is also disturbed.

Eating slowly, being aware of the food, savoring its taste, texture, and aroma are critically important in restoring the act of eating to a manageable physical function. The following checklist will help you assess your child's eating style. After each item, check the appropriate column.

	Often	Sometimes	Never
Gulps down breakfast and runs out to school or to catch a bus.			

	Often	Sometimes	Never
Eats as if ravenously hungry.			
Thinks and talks about un- pleasant, irritating, or stressful events while eating.			
During mealtimes, dis- cusses important matters that require making a difficult decision.			
Rushes in from playing and sits down panting to eat meal.			

If you checked "Often" or "Sometimes" for two or more items, chances are that the process of mealtime eating could use some attention. A few changes in the mealtime environment can have an important impact on your child's eating style.

There are three things you can do to help your child to eat slowly and learn when to stop. The first is the timing of your meals. In the morning, start breakfast at an earlier time so as not to crowd the tardy bell at school. If your child has a problem getting up and getting started in the morning, simply announce the rules and stick by them. If your child does not come to breakfast when it is scheduled to start, then he doesn't eat any breakfast at all. That means no quick bite and nothing to eat on the way to school. The following morning you will wake him or her up a bit earlier. Having no breakfast at all will not hurt your child for a day or two while you are affirming the rule that breakfast must be eaten properly. The evening meal might also have to be rescheduled so that everyone has time to slow down and relax a few minutes before starting to eat.

The second task is to establish a quiet, pleasant atmosphere for eating. Get rid of all competing attractions, especially the television and radio. Discourage telephone calls by asking anyone who calls to wait until after mealtime. Talk about pleasant things only. The discipline this may require is well worth the effort.

The third step is to teach your child some new ways of behavior. You teach by example and by explanation. The example you set will profoundly influence the way your child eats although the effects of this influence may not be immediate. The best example you can set is to be relaxed when you eat. Pause for a few seconds before picking up your knife and fork. Check your facial muscles and the muscles in your arms and across your shoulders. Release all the tension you feel and let those muscles relax. Chew your food slowly. Comment on how good it smells and how nice it looks, even if this means praising your own cooking. Part way through the meal, stop eating for as long as two or three minutes. Relax again. Talk about something interesting. Before you resume eating, check your own body cues and decide whether you really want more.

After you have improved your own eating, you can start helping your child slow down by telling him or her how to do the same things you have done. If the child asks "why?" you can say that eating slowly helps you enjoy the food. It helps the body start the digestion process, it gives the body a chance to signal when it has received enough food, and it improves your chances of becoming aware of that message. Eating this way also makes you a more pleasant person and a more enjoyable companion at mealtimes.

9. Eating on Schedule

It's easier to do something every day when you're on a schedule that doesn't change much. This applies to eating meals, too. Many overweight children come from homes in which mealtimes are unpredictable. In some cases the whole family waits to have dinner until the working parent comes home, and particularly with office jobs, that time can fluctuate quite a bit from day to day. In other cases, the parent who does the cooking changes around the child's mealtimes to suit the child—if he wants to go to an early movie, he's allowed to have dinner later; if she wants to go visit a friend, she's given her dinner early. And in yet other cases, children get away with skipping a meal altogether if they'd rather be off doing something else. The more that mealtimes are unpredictable, the more difficult it will be for your child to acquire good regular eating habits. The child gets the idea that when you eat isn't very important, and consequently that *how often* you eat as well as *what* you eat can't be too important, either.

The task of scheduling meals and making certain that your children stick to the schedule won't be easy, until you decide that it's important and, through your actions, convince your children that you mean it. After a while, your children will begin to plan their activities so that they don't conflict with dinnertime, instead of vice versa. You may have to make some changes in your own activities, too, so that you're not interfering with the schedule. Having said this, however, we should emphasize that you can maintain some flexibility. If you normally serve dinner at 6:30 but have to work late on Fridays, fine: On Fridays, schedule dinner for 7:30. If the working parent can never predict exactly when he or she will be home, schedule the dinner late enough so that the family can eat together at least four out of five days a week. And don't allow children to skip meals. You may think that a fat child will benefit by not consuming those calories, but nine times out of ten the child will more than make up for it later by eating candy and rich snacks to satisfy the hunger that should have been satisfied by a balanced meal.

We've already talked about eating breakfast and controlling snacks. Both of these go a long way toward putting your child's eating on schedule. Now all you need to do is schedule lunch, dinner, and perhaps one other minimeal or "scheduled" snack. When your child gets home from school may be an opportune time for a scheduled snack. This snack can be appetizing and nutritious and it can include energy (protein and nonsugar carbohydrates) that will sustain him until dinnertime.

Another advantage of eating on schedule is that it makes it easier to convince children that those times of the day should be devoted to eating and social conversation—and nothing else. When children watch television or read or listen to music while eating, it's easy for them to hardly notice what or how much they're eating. If their attention is on an exciting TV car chase while they're eating dessert, they may suddenly look down and discover all the dessert is gone and they haven't had any enjoyment from it. Naturally they then ask for a second helping. A quiet, relaxed meal lets children see, smell, and taste their food and allows them to pay attention when their bodies tell them they've had enough. And there's a bonus: It regularly brings the family together in a pleasant atmosphere.

When you've established a mealtime schedule, your child will develop a cycle of hunger that corresponds to mealtimes. When this occurs he or she will be less likely to feel hungry between meals, and you both will have achieved an important step in the control of eating behavior. To see whether this is a behavior you need to change, put a check in the "Yes" or "No" columns following. If you check the "Yes" column twice or more, you should plan to work on this behavior.

	YES	NO
1. Do your mealtimes vary from day to day?		
2. Do your child's activities often interfere with his or her mealtimes?		
3. Does your child skip a meal at least once a week?		
4. Does your child often do something else (like watching TV) while eating?		
5. Are mealtimes in your house hectic rather than relaxed?		

10. Learning About Food and Exercise

You may remember we said earlier that the important thing is establishing good eating and exercise habits and that you needn't explain what you're doing unless your child is curious. This is especially true with very young children and when first starting a program. At the beginning your kids will be likely to argue with any explanation you give, simply because they automatically resist changes. But as the child gets older, he or she will be eating fewer meals at home and will have a lot more choice about food and exercise. To some extent, the good habits you have helped your son or daughter to acquire will persist. For example, it's rare for someone who is used to a good nourishing breakfast to give up that habit. Even so, habit combined with understanding is stronger than habit alone. For this reason you should make sure that as your child gets older, he or she learns the basis of nutrition and exercise. With this knowledge, the child will know how to stay healthy and fit even when his or her lifestyle changes.

Some schools do an excellent job of teaching students about food and exercise; a great many do not. In any event, you should support this kind of knowledge in the home, which means you may have to get a couple of books out of your public library and do a bit of studying yourself. Magazines like *Reader's Digest* and *Family Circle* often have articles about health, and your newspaper probably does, too. If you clip these articles and save them, you'll soon find you have your own library.

How much your child is ready to understand about these topics will depend upon his or her intellectual maturity. As a rough guide, the following is the way that Harvard professor of nutrition Dr. Jean Mayer feels nutritional education should be broken down.

School Grades	Topics
1, 2, 3	The many different kinds of food available Regional and ethnic foods Plants and animals used as foods Where milk comes from How butter is made How wheat grows and how it is milled Fishing and the history of food
4, 5, 6	The body and how it functions How food is carried to the cells How food is turned into fuel for the body How the body uses this fuel How the organs of the body work
7, 8, 9	Nutrition—the role of carbohydrates, fats, proteins, minerals, vitamins How to read the nutritional and ingredient labels on packaged food
10, 11, 12	Physical fitness and weight control What calories are Protein and amino acids—animal and vegetable sources Vitamins and the prevention of disease

Take a moment to check off which of these topics you think your child knows about. If there are gaps, you can plan to help your boy or girl understand those points yourself, or encourage him or her to take related courses in school. We suggest you make this effort after your child has made a good start toward establishing the other eating and exercise behaviors discussed in this chapter.

Chapter Summary

There are ten eating and exercise behaviors that account for the weight problems of most obese children. You can judge to what extent your child has trouble with each behavior, and learn how to teach them to your child. They are: 1. Eating a good breakfast; 2. Controlling snacks; 3. Controlling calories; 4. Eating balanced meals; 5. Keeping food in its place; 6. Getting enough exercise; 7. Easing tension; 8. Eating slowly; 9. Eating on schedule; 10. Learning about food and exercise. The next chapters will tell you exactly how to work these ten behaviors into a program that will make your child slimmer and more fit.

6

The Psychology of Healthful Eating and Exercise

If you've ever tried to change any of your own habits, you're well aware that knowing what to do and doing it are two different things. It's easy to acknowledge that smoking is bad for you and that you should stop, but losing the habit can be a nightmare. Similarly, most overweight people know that the way to lose weight is to eat less and exercise more, but most of us can only manage that for a few weeks before going back to our old ways.

Fortunately, in the last twenty years, and especially in the last five years, scientists and researchers have found out a lot about how habits are formed and how they can be broken. Not surprisingly, habits have more to do with our minds than our bodies. The psychological addiction to overeating is stronger than the bodily addiction. So in order to help your child develop and maintain good eating habits, you should be aware of a few psychological facts. With these facts and techniques, you will be able to painlessly change the habits that have made your child overweight. We begin with some general principles or rules, which lead to a description of incentives and how to apply them in changing specific behaviors.

RULE A:

Don't give up your responsibility to influence your children's behavior.

This rule will sound ridiculously obvious to some parents. Yet a lot of parents have given up their responsibility to do what is best for their children if the children object. Here's an example, from a recent *Newsweek* article about television's influence on children:

And few parents can cope with its tyrannical allure. Recently, Dr. Benjamin Spock brought his stepdaughter and granddaughter to New York for a tour of the Bronx Zoo and the Museum of Modern Art. But the man who has the prescription for everything from diaper rash to bed-wetting could not dislodge the kids from their hotel room. "I couldn't get them away from the goddamned TV set," recalls Spock. "It made me sick."

It is enough to make you sick. But the question is why blame television when the responsibility for turning the set on and off lies with the parent? Television *is* guilty, however, of fostering this image of the abdicated parent, especially in commercials. For example, a laundry detergent ad shows a distressed mother trying to cope with a child who has just happily covered her new outfit with mud. The mother seems to conclude, "There's nothing I can do to prevent my child from getting dirty. Thank goodness I have Brand X detergent!" Another ad shows a boy tracking dirt across the kitchen floor. The poor mother's response is, "I can't possibly teach my child to take his muddy boots off at the door. All I can do is use Brand X floor cleaner to scrub the floor behind him."

Television programs themselves rarely realistically reflect family life. If a problem is shown, it has to be resolved within 30 or 60 minutes. If the program is a situation comedy, the adversity is used as a source of humor, and at the end everyone gets together for a wholesome fade-out, chuckling and living happily ever after. Programs like "All in the Family" changed this pattern a bit: Formerly, topics such as alcoholism were never mentioned; now they're allowed, but dealt with in a superficial and often insincere way. The dramatic programs are interested mainly in people who are murderers, victims, relatives of either, and detectives and policemen. If you believe the comedies, you conclude people don't really have problems. If you believe the dramas you conclude people have so many problems that they continually stab, shoot, or strangle each other.

Television can be a wonderful source of entertainment and information. The difficulty is that people watch it indiscriminately, almost constantly, and to the exclusion of most other activities. Consciously, or subconsciously, they compare themselves to the characters they see, and if their values are different from the values of the people on TV, they feel guilty. Children instinctively exploit this. They may even say, "The Mommy on TV didn't yell at *her* daughter when she tracked mud into the kitchen!" Or, "Why shouldn't I get to ride a motorcycle and wear a leather jacket? Fonzie does."

The easiest thing for the parent to do is to give in and

give up. If you do, the child is the one who pays the consequence. For the moment, he or she will be grateful, for example, for being given endless snacks, for being allowed to skip breakfast, for not being encouraged to exercise. Only when the child is mature enough to realize the penalties of being overweight will he or she begin to wonder. "Didn't Mom and Dad care enough about me to prevent this?"

Buying this book reflects your concern for your children. The techniques we'll be discussing through the rest of the book let you influence your children's behavior without becoming a tyrant and without having to rely on punishment to bring about the necessary changes. It's important that you remember that what you are doing is accepting the responsibility of parenthood. Not only is that still possible, it's praiseworthy—even if it seems to have gone out of fashion.

RULE B:

Don't discourage your child's enjoyment of food.

This may come as a surprise to you, but many overweight people actually don't enjoy food very much. The usual picture of the obese person is that of someone who loves all kinds of food and spends long hours cooking and then enjoying meals. Yet almost the opposite is true. The average overweight person eats a small *number* of foods, but he or she eats those particular foods in large quantities. These foods are usually fairly boring ones. Either they are relatively bland: potatoes, bread, butter;

or they are very sweet: chocolate, candy bars, jams, and jellies. The overweight person tends to eat on the run, to gulp down the meal, and to pay little attention to the more subtle aspects of food.

As well as taste, food can appeal to the senses of sight, sound, smell, and touch. With regard to taste, separate taste buds on the tongue respond to substances that are sweet, sour, and bitter. Food comes in many colors and shapes for aesthetic appeal to our eyes. The most distinctive food sound is the crunching of crisp, raw carrots, lettuce, apples, and the like. Also the cooking sounds of sizzling steaks or bubbling soups are pleasant because they are associated with the eating soon to follow. Likewise, the aroma of food is usually strongest while food is in preparation, especially while cooking or baking. And finally, food comes in a variety of textures, from liquid to solid, coarse to smooth, and soft to hard. The sense of touch also responds to the temperature of the food. The combination of the stimulation of all the senses makes eating one of the pleasures of life.

Another attraction of eating is that it's often linked with social activity. Taking someone to dinner or sharing a meal at home makes eating a more pleasant activity because the enjoyment of the food is enhanced by the enjoyment of each other's company. Family dinners can be a pleasant occasion for exchanging information and viewpoints. Overweight people often lose out on this enjoyment. They may be too ashamed of their eating habits to relish eating in public, or they may be so anxious to bolt down their food that there isn't time for relaxed conversation.

Urging you to encourage your child to enjoy food may sound like a recipe for disaster. Won't it make him or her want to eat even more? The answer is no. When your child learns to enjoy the many qualities of food (not just taste), he or she will select a greater variety of food. This will provide a greater range of nutrients and thus a more balanced diet.

Mi Ae Lipe, the six-year-old daughter of one of the authors, chooses carrots when offered both carrots and cookies on a plate. She likes the bright orange color of the carrots, their crunchiness, and their mildly sweet taste. She also knows that the sugar in cookies makes holes in your teeth, and she's proud of her beautiful white teeth and the fact that she's never had a cavity.

It's also true that as your child enjoys food more, he or she will eat more slowly to extend the pleasure, and by eating more slowly will tend to eat less.

The way you can encourage this enjoyment is to serve a limited quantity of a large variety of foods in the course of a week. This can be as simple as switching to a different kind of salad dressing once in a while, or serving a variety of vegetables instead of the usual peas and carrots. Some nights, cheese, fruit, and crackers can serve as dessert. At first this may be resisted by your son or daughter (and maybe even by your spouse). Don't insist that your children finish everything on their plates, but praise them for trying the new food. When you do serve something different, you can talk a bit about what it is, where it grows, and what it tastes like. After an initial show of resistance the child's curiosity will usually win out.

RULE C:

Encourage change in small, easy steps.

Reasonable people accept that it takes a while to master a behavior such as playing the guitar or driving a car or reading. But the same people are sometimes indignant that it also takes a while to change eating and exercise habits and thereby lose weight. These people would laugh if you offered them pills and said, "Here, take these and in four weeks you'll be able to play the piano"; but collectively they spend millions of dollars on "miracle" diets and "miracle" diet books. The only miracle is that every year they spend more on such pie-in-the-sky products. The inescapable fact is that successful behavior change usually comes about slowly. There is a fitting Chinese proverb: "The journey of a thousand miles begins with a single step."

It's important not to expect too much of your child all at once. In Chapter Eight you'll find out how to go about selecting the first step and the next and the next. Each new behavior to be encouraged must represent a small enough change so that your child is virtually assured of success. Even one small success is a step forward. It gives you and your child more self-confidence in taking the next step, and eventually you will find you have arrived at the end of the journey to fitness and good health.

RULE D:

Use praise instead of criticism to change behavior.

It has been shown over and over again that criticizing

bad eating habits doesn't lead to their improvement. In fact, many times it makes things worse. There are several reasons for this. In the first place, children want attention from their parents. They even prefer criticism to no attention at all. If you make a big deal out of your child's overeating, that puts your child in the spotlight, and he or she will repeat that behavior again to get more attention. This can be especially true when there are several children in the family; one may use his or her eating habits to be the center of attention at mealtimes. The result isn't a good one. The child builds a negative view of himself or herself and earns the resentment of the other children.

Secondly, constant criticism makes mealtimes less pleasant for the whole family and is likely to make everyone more inclined to gulp down his food and skip a meal when possible.

Finally, being in the position of nagging your child makes you feel guilty and unhappy and may lead you to decide that trying to change your boy's or girl's eating habits isn't worth the effort.

As we've just indicated, you child wants your attention. If you respond to bad behavior, it will increase. If you respond to good behavior, *that* will increase. So instead of looking for things to criticize, you must look for things to praise. This could be difficult at first, and you may have to compliment something small: Perhaps your child took only two helpings instead of his usual three, or perhaps you were able to get him to have a piece of toast in the morning instead of going off to school on an empty stomach.

Naturally there are common-sense limits to exchanging criticism for praise. If little Bobby dumps his plate of spinach over little Wendy's head, you'd still be expected to give him some pretty vehement criticism, rather than saying, "Wasn't it good of Bobby not to break the plate as he hit Wendy with it." But in less drastic situations, a steady and consistent program of praising good eating and exercise related behaviors will soon pay off.

The source of this rule is a psychological principle: *Rewarded behavior occurs again.* Praise is one kind of reward, or incentive.

RULE E:

Recognize and use the power of the incentives.

For generations the incentive of desserts has been used successfully to teach children to eat all the food on their plates. This has been called "grandma's law." Grandma usually put it like this:

"First clean up your plate. Then you may have dessert."

Unfortunately this sometimes had the effect of training children to eat more than they wanted or needed, which goes to show how powerful it is. It's not just grandmas who use incentives, it's parents, teachers, doctors, and all adults who deal with children successfully. Let's look at one example:

Mrs. Alexander was irritated by her eight-year-old boy's habit of wetting his bed. Her doctor could find no medical reason for this problem. Whenever her son wet the bed, he woke up and yelled for help. Mrs. Alexander would then get up, bathe him, give him clean pyjamas and bedding, reassure him, and tuck him in.

Mrs. Alexander was unintentionally rewarding her son for wetting his bed. When he did it, he received more concern and loving attention than at almost any other time. When she realized this, Mrs. Alexander switched things around so that he'd be rewarded for staying dry. She told her son, "From now on, don't wake me up when you wet your bed. Get up, wash yourself, change your pyjamas and sheets. But when you stay dry, I'll come in in the morning and we'll read a story before you get up."

The first few nights her son continued to wet the bed and found that his mother meant what she said. The morning after his first dry night, she praised him profusely and spent an extra fifteen minutes reading a story to him.

As we will discuss in detail a little later, an incentive can also be a tangible thing, like a box of crayons or a new dress or a toy. Occasionally someone will object that this is "bribery" and that children should behave well on general principles. This reflects a poor understanding of human behavior. After all, why do you work 40 hours a week? Because work is good, or because you have the incentive of a paycheck at the end of the week? Why do you try to look your best when you attend a social event? Because there is some absolute good in looking attractive, or because you hope that others will admire your looks? The range of incentives is very wide: You may do something because you hope it'll earn you a thousand dollars or because you hope it'll contribute to world peace. The more sophisticated and advanced we become, the more we strive for unselfish and longer term goals. Children, however, aren't sophisticated and respond better to immediate rewards, whether it be a hug from Dad or a comic book. There is nothing immoral about using incentives to bring about good behavior. Also, once a new behavior is established, you can phase out the incentive and attach it to the next good behavior you want your child to master.

RULE F:

Use anything your child wants as an incentive.

As you read the previous rule, you may have started wondering what could serve as an incentive for your child. The answer is: anything your child wants that isn't destructive or harmful. We've already seen that you shouldn't use food as a reward, but there are lots of alternatives. It could be staying up late, watching a television show, being taken to the movies, being allowed to borrow the car, and so forth. Obviously the age of the child will affect the nature of the incentive as will the child's current likes and dislikes. We've already briefly touched upon praise as an incentive, but we'd like to expand on that because it is one of the most reliable rewards, and it's free. First, here are a couple of examples of how teachers have used praise to shape children's behavior:

Miss Bigby was a kindergarten teacher whose class was one of the best behaved and seemingly happiest of any class anywhere. One approach in particular seemed to stand out as a factor in the effective learning environment created by Miss Bigby. Whenever the class started to get restless, for example just before recess, Miss Bigby would look around the room for some child who was working quietly. Then she would say, "I like the way Tommy is reading his book." The other students then tended to imitate the student who was being praised.

Here's an example of how a teacher used praise to shape the behavior of older children:

Mrs. Tipton was a small woman with a soft voice. She felt intimidated by her aggressive sixth-grade class and tended to be on the look-out for undesirable behavior. The level of activity, confusion, and noise was usually quite high in her classroom and she could often be heard shouting commands for the students to "STOP IT!" This is the kind of trap into which any adult can easily fall. One day the school's principal, Mrs. Leonetti, sat in Mrs. Tipton's class and counted the number of praise statements that Mrs. Tipton made. She suggested that Mrs. Tipton quadruple the number of praise statements and also stop yelling at the students. Mrs. Tipton made a point of finding at least one student's behavior to praise every 15 or 20 minutes. She would praise the class or a student in the class for doing something right, no matter how small or seemingly insignificant the good behavior was. The result was rather astounding to Mrs. Tipton. The students' behavior still wasn't perfect, of course, but it did improve considerably and rapidly. Furthermore as the students came to associate Mrs. Tipton with something they found pleasant (praise) rather than something unpleasant (constant shouting), they grew to like her better and to respond more positively to her teaching.

Praise is time-honored and universally effective. When a child is frequently praised, the occasions when he or she is reprimanded are all the more effective. The child quickly learns to discriminate between what is acceptable behavior and what is not.

The more potential incentives you have at your disposal, the more impact you will have upon your child's eating behavior. In Chapter Seven, we'll make some further specific suggestions regarding incentives to use with your child. First, there are two rules about using incentives effectively.

RULE G:

Reward action, not promises.

It doesn't work to give a reward now for something you want your child to do later. An incentive given before the act is no longer an incentive. It doesn't work, for example, to let a child watch his favorite television program at 1:00 P.M. on the promise that he will take only one helping of potatoes at supper time. It would be far better to let the program serve as a reward for desirable eating behavior that occurred at lunch. A parent might say, for example, "You took only one helping of potatoes at lunch. I'm proud of you. You may watch your television program now if you want to. If you do as well at supper, I'll play a game of checkers with you afterward, if you'd like."

Rewards are most effective if they are given soon after the good behavior. As adults, we have learned to work for far-away rewards. We may save money all year for a vacation, for example. But for children even a week's delay can seem an eternity, and the prospect of a small reward in half an hour is more appealing than the promise of a large reward in a month.

RULE H:

Be very clear about what you expect of your child.

If you tell your child that you'll give a reward if he or she "cuts down on snacks," you may find that he or she eats one bite less of a candy bar and assumes that this should be considered a success. (There's a certain age at which all children act as though they're going to grow up to be lawyers.) The way to prevent such misunderstandings is to be specific: The reward will be given if the child eats nothing between lunch' and dinner, for example. Similarly, telling your child to eat more slowly can be too general. Instead you could suggest that the child swallow each bite before taking the next one, and rest his or her hands on the table while chewing, instead of having the next forkful hovering in midair like an airliner waiting to land.

These eight rules, based on principles of psychology and behavior change, will help you to ease the transformation of your child's eating and exercise habits.

Chapter Summary

Knowing which of your child's behaviors need to be changed is crucial. Knowing how to bring about this change is equally important. Psychologists recently have discovered a lot about how to teach new behaviors, and from their research, we have developed eight rules:

1) Don't give up your responsibility to influence your child's behavior.
2) Don't discourage your child's enjoyment of food.
3) Encourage change in the form of small, easy steps.
4) Use praise instead of criticism to change behavior.
5) Recognize and use the power of incentives.
6) Use anything your child wants as an incentive.
7) Reward action, not promises.
8) Be very clear about what you expect of your child.

These rules will all come into use in Chapter Eight, when you will develop a behavior-change program for your child.

7

Incentives to Use With Your Child

What's a good incentive? In the last chapter you found out that almost anything your child wants to have or do can be an incentive. You probably have at least some ideas about incentives to use with your child. After all, most kids spend a lot of time buttonholing their parents and talking about what they want.

In case your child is shy or seems to want only material things like toys, we're going to describe ten nonmaterialistic incentives. They work and they don't cost anything. It's also important to understand how to use these incentives in a practical way. After reading the five case studies at the end of this chapter, you'll see how incentives have been used to get kids to eat breakfast, cut down on snacks, and change other behaviors. It should give you some good ideas about how to use incentives with your child. Which of these incentives would motivate your son or daughter:

Crawling into Bed with Their Parents

Young children love to do this because it gives them a sense of security and warmth. This may not appeal to you as a Monday morning practice, when summoning up the stamina to get up wouldn't be made any easier by having a tiny voice pleading to hear the story of Goldilocks for the forty-fifth time that month. It may work out, however, if Saturday or Sunday morning is a lazy time when you all enjoy staying in bed for a few minutes longer.

Playing with a Friend

By definition a friend is someone with whom your child enjoys spending time. One of the questions you hear most often is "May I go play with . . . ?" We're not suggesting that you make your child's social life totally dependent upon his or her eating or exercise behaviors, but you can use this incentive selectively. For example, you may say, "Yes, after you've finished mowing the lawn" (exercise behavior), or "Yes, if you eat slowly, the way I've shown you" (eating behavior).

Sleeping Late or Getting up Early

There are night people and day people. The bodily rhythms which make you one or the other are already operating in children. Obviously children have to establish a routine that gives them the right amount of sleep and gets them off to school on time, but especially on weekends you can give them a bit of leeway. Some children will appreciate the chance to sleep late. Others will enjoy not being yelled at if they feel like starting the day an hour before the rest of the family can pry open their eyelids. For the latter type, you may want to lay out a selection of books or toys with which the child will be allowed to play whenever he or she feels like waking up. If you're a late sleeper, the line-up of toys should not include drums, dolls that speak above a whisper, or model tanks and cars with realistic-sounding motors.

Wearing a Favorite Shirt or Dress

Children often have a favorite item of clothing which they are allowed to wear only on special occasions. You can make a special occasion of your child's success in changing one of his or her behaviors. Not only does this give the child enjoyment, but also a sense of pride in his or her accomplishment.

Watching Television or Going to a Movie

The notion that watching television is a privilege, rather than a right or an automatic habit like breathing, has gone out of fashion. You can revive it by taking control of the on and off switch of your set, especially if you have younger children. How many shootings, stabbings, chokings, rapes, shootouts, and fistfights does your six year old see in an average evening of viewing? Count them sometime and see if it's not too many. How many other activities is your child missing by watching one after another inane situation comedy? If you have established the idea that watching TV is one of many activities (like reading, solving puzzles, learning to play a musical instrument, playing games, and developing some athletic skill), then being allowed to watch a particular TV program can serve as a strong incentive for your child.

Older children will also respond to the incentive of going to a movie with you or on their own. Movie theaters are dark, comfortable places where a child can escape from any demands or interruptions for a couple of hours. The biggest danger is the candy counter, which sells the worst kinds of candy at double the usual price. One solution is to provide your child with some nonfattening snacks to take along, or to buy the least offensive of the snack foods usually offered, unbuttered popcorn.

Staying up Late

For some children the chance to stay up even 10 or 15 minutes later than their usual bedtime can be very rewarding. This can also be used if they want to see a suitable television program that is on a bit later than they are used to staying up, or if friends of the family or relatives are visiting. For teenagers, a variation of this is letting them stay out a half hour later than usual when they go out with friends.

Talking to a Friend on the Telephone

As children move toward and through the teenage years, this can become an obsession rather than just an activity. Naturally you will want to let your child maintain normal social contacts and make brief calls whenever necessary. However, for the sake of your budget and your relationships with friends who may actually want to call *you* (a possibility which most teenagers regard as pure fantasy), you'll probably want to let your child conduct marathon phone conversations only as an occasional privilege.

Performing for an Audience

Younger children delight in being the center of attention, but parents can't always oblige. Therefore one good incentive is promising to be the audience for 10 minutes while your child puts on a performance of some kind: a puppet show, a series of riddles or jokes, imitations of the characters on Sesame Street, a rendition of "Old Mac-Donald Had a Farm," a dance, or whatever your budding performer chooses. This has the added benefit of encouraging your child to use his or her imagination and can be a useful way of encouraging shy children to feel more at ease.

Reading or Having a Story Read

Reading to a young child is one way of encouraging him or her to appreciate the written word. It's also another time when your child is able to have your undivided attention. As the child gets older, the promise of having you read a bedtime story to him or her can be replaced by the promise of being allowed to read to you for 15 minutes before the light is turned out. For children who enjoy reading, the promise of being bought a book they want or being taken to the library are also good incentives.

Playing a Game with You

Children enjoy competing with adults when there's a chance they can win. Since adults seem so powerful, it's good for kids to have the opportunity to triumph over Mom or Dad once in a while. The best games are those in which chance determines the outcome, rather than ones in which you have to deliberately play badly to let the child win (a child is sharper than a Las Vegas dealer at spotting a rigged game, and it makes him or her feel even more powerless, to realize that victory is possible only if Mom or Dad lets it happen).

Now that you've seen some of the incentives available, let's look at how some parents have put them to work in changing specific behaviors.

CASE STUDY: Eliminating Candy

Mr. and Mrs. Camden wanted their daughter Roberta to keep her beautiful white teeth free of cavities and to avoid the other dangers of eating too much candy. They didn't keep candy around the house and only occasionally served sweet desserts. One incentive they used was praise: They praised Roberta for brushing her teeth and for taking moderate helpings when sweet foods were served.

They also appealed to Roberta's pride in her own appearance by complimenting her pretty teeth and her clear skin and they made sure she was aware that eating too much candy wouldn't be good for either. When Roberta started school, they showed her how to refuse candy politely without offending the offerer. If the other person insisted, she was to take it and bring it home to be thrown away. Roberta never built up an addiction to sweets because her parents gave her a balanced diet, informed her of the drawbacks of candy, and never used food as a substitute for love or attention. By using the rewards of praise and pride in her appearance, they ensured that Roberta didn't lose her good eating habits as she grew older.

CASE STUDY: Eating Breakfast

Margie was a high school freshman who was about 30 pounds overweight. She'd been overweight most of her life but was finding it especially troublesome now because it led to a very poor social life. One of her habits was sleeping late and skipping breakfast—in fact, she assumed she was doing herself a favor by skipping a meal. Margie's parents, who were also overweight, had learned that a good breakfast reduces snacking and lets you cut down on the quantity of food eaten at lunch and dinner. But they also recognized that Margie was at an age when she wanted more independence. If they tried to force her to eat breakfast, she would almost automatically resist. Instead, they used independence as a reward. In return for eating breakfast with her parents over a certain period of time, Margie was allowed to make various decisions about her own life. These varied from week to week: from choosing her own clothing, to deciding which evenings she would go out, to being allowed to stay out later on weekends. As well as eventually learning to enjoy eating breakfast, she also felt a greater maturity as a result of her evolving independence.

CASE STUDY: Exercising

Roger was a plump nine-year-old bookworm. He had come to avoid exercise whenever possible because he was teased about his lack of coordination and his lack of stamina at games. His usual routine was to come home from school, fix himself a huge snack and settle down with a science fiction book until dinnertime. He also continually pestered his parents for money with which to buy the latest science fiction magazines. Roger's mother wanted him to exercise so he would lose weight and develop a healthier, stronger body. From her doctor, she got a booklet describing an exercise program that started slowly and very gradually became more demanding. Roger's mother decided to use his love of reading as an incentive. She bought a calendar and posted it on the kitchen bulletin board. When Roger came home from school he did his exercises, and then was allowed to put an "X" on that day's date. If there were at least five X's at the end of the week, his mother bought him a science fiction magazine when she went shopping on Saturdays. If not, Roger was turned down in his requests for money with which to buy the magazines. After making sure his parents really meant what they said, he settled into his exercise routine. He never turned into an athlete, but as he became fitter, he was teased less and stopped trying to avoid participating in his P.E. classes.

CASE STUDY: Controlling Evening Snacks

One reason twelve-year-old Cynthia was so overweight was that she ate snacks almost continuously between suppertime and her bedtime. She filled up on chips and dip, ice cream, cookies, and practically anything else she could find. At first her parents tried to cope with the problem by not buying this junk food. Cynthia responded by making sandwiches, drinking glass after glass of milk, and even eating cold leftovers. Her parents assumed this insatiable hunger must be a sign of a physical disease, but the family doctor's examination showed no physical problems. Finally her parents realized that her snacking was much worse on evenings when she had homework. She seemed to be using eating as a way of postponing homework or escaping the difficult parts. Cynthia's parents did two things. First, they found out which parts of her homework were most difficult for her and (with the agreement of her teacher) helped her with those. Her teacher also made a special effort to make sure Cynthia understood the homework assignments and praised her when her homework was done correctly. Secondly, her parents worked out an agreement that Cynthia could have only one snack per evening and not until 8:00 P.M. But on evenings when she had homework she could have her snack as soon as she had finished her homework, even if it was before 8:00. At first she rushed through her home-work doing a sloppy job, but her parents sent her back to her desk to do it over. Gradually she discovered she could get her homework done more quickly and better by con-centrating on it, rather than by jumping up and eating every time she encountered a problem. Because the eating had been caused by anxiety, she ate less as the anxiety of doing homework was reduced.

CASE STUDY: Eating Slowly

Ten-year-old Freddie had developed the habit of shoveling down his food as quickly as possible. He wasn't in a hurry to go somewhere or do something, he just assumed that the faster he ate, the more he could get. His figure revealed that his logic was correct. His parents were upset by his weight problem and were embarrassed by Freddie's eating habits when guests came to dinner. Reminders to eat more slowly seemed to work for about a minute; then Freddie's machinelike arm was back in action. His father finally decided to try to use incentives to slow Freddie down. He and Freddie prepared a list of things Freddie wanted to have or to do: to go to a certain horror film, to spend a night at his best friend's house, to buy a particular comic book, to pitch his tent in the back-yard and sleep out there for a night, and so on. Next, his father demonstrated how Freddie was to eat: to sit up straight, take a moderate-sized bite of food, rest his hand on the table while he chewed and swallowed, and then take another bite. For the next two weeks each morning before breakfast Freddie picked an incentive for that day.

He would not be reminded by anyone how he should eat, but if he ate breakfast and dinner as he had been shown, he would receive his reward after dinner. Freddie missed out on two days the first week, and only one day the second week. For the next month, Freddie picked a larger incentive, but had to eat properly for a whole week to earn the incentive. By the end of the month, the new behavior had become a habit. Because he ate more slowly, he ate less and was beginning to lose weight. Freddie's father, pleased with the success of the incentive plan, phased out the rewards for this behavior (they were no longer needed) and switched to using incentives to change another of Freddie's poor eating habits.

These five episodes demonstrate how incentives are a natural part of the behavior-change process. Children feel a sense of accomplishment when they earn their privileges, rather than being handed them. In this way, the use of incentives also helps children to mature and develop a sense of responsibility. The next chapter brings together all the material you've read so far and the information you've jotted down in this book. The final thing you should do before you can develop a behavior-change program for your child is to jot down on the next page the incentives you feel will work with your child. Some of them will be the same as ones we have mentioned, others will derive from your unique knowledge of your child. Try to come up with at least a dozen.

INCENTIVES TO USE

1.

2.

3.

4.

5.

6.

7.

8.

9.

10.

11.

12.

Chapter Summary

Anything your child wants or enjoys doing can be an incentive you use to encourage good eating and exercise habits. Among the incentives parents have found to be particularly effective are:

Playing with a friend
Wearing a favorite shirt or dress
Staying up late
Crawling into bed with their parents
Sleeping late or getting up early
Performing for an audience
Watching television or going to a movie
Reading or having a story read
Playing a game with you
Talking to a friend on the telephone

Incentives like these can be used to establish various behaviors: eliminating candy from the diet, eating breakfast, exercising, controlling snacks, and chewing food slowly, among others. Although this chapter will have given you some ideas about incentives to use, your own knowledge of your child's likes and dislikes will suggest additional ones.

8

Designing a Program for Your Child

The time has come to apply many of the things you have learned and the information you have gathered in the course of reading the previous chapters. To be really effective, any behavior-change program has to be individualized. That is, it has to match the needs and characteristics of the individual whose behavior is supposed to be changed. With the knowledge you now have about why your child is overweight, the importance of good nutrition and exercise, the most important behaviors related to eating and weight, and the use of incentives, you're ready to design a program to fit your child. We'll show you how to do it, step-by-step.

STEP 1: Record Your Child's Weight

To find your child's starting weight, you should do more than simply weigh him or her once. Weight changes from day to day and even from hour to hour, and not all these variations are related to what's eaten. For example, we are all lighter in the mornings than in the evenings, partly because we breathe out a lot of moisture while we sleep. Weigh your child once a day for two weeks, at about the same time each day. Record the weight on the blank two-week weight chart. Write down your child's weight on the first day. Each following day put a dot on the position matching the day of the week and the amount of weight your child has gained or lost. We've included a sample chart completed by Laura R. for her ten-year-old daughter Susan. As you can see, on the second day, Susan weighed half a pound more than on the first. On the third day, she weighed about a quarter of a pound less than on the previous day. At the end of the two weeks Laura drew lines connecting all the dots. This shows the trend of Susan's weight. Although the line is jagged, its general direction is upward. We can see that not only did Susan start this two-week period at a weight level above the range recommended for her age and height, but she is continuing to gain weight. If the line is level, the child is remaining at his or her weight, if the line points downward, the youngster is already losing weight.

Don't make changes in your child's eating habits during this two-week weighing period. Rather, use the time to plan the entire program. Then you will have an accurate figure of your child's weight, and the trend of his or her weight before you begin the program. Soon you will be comparing your child's progress against these figures.

STEP 2: Decide on a Weight Goal for Your Child

Because we are all different in so many ways, it's impossible to say that a person who is so tall should weigh

SAMPLE WEIGHT CHART FOR SUSAN R.

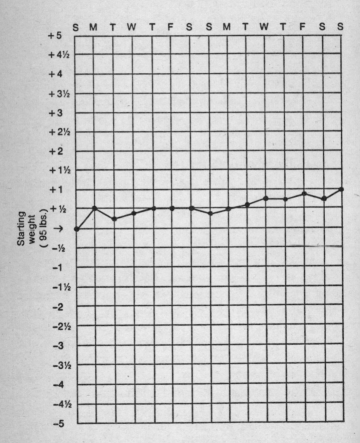

1: TWO-WEEK WEIGHT CHART FOR YOUR CHILD

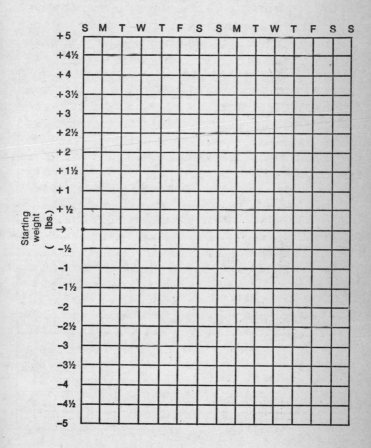

exactly so many pounds. We have provided weight tables that indicate the approximate weights for boys and girls of different ages and another of suggested weights for different heights. *These are intended as rough guidelines only.* Use them in conjunction with your own judgment to come up with a weight goal for your child. Don't try to transform a very fat child into a very thin one—settle for an average weight. Try to figure out at what point the other children will stop asking, "Hey kid, how come you're so fat?" That will be your goal. Write it down at the top of Chart 2.

STEP 3: Rank Your Child's Problem Behaviors

In Chapter Six you read about ten eating-related behaviors and thought about whether each one applies to your child. We'd like you to quickly review that chapter and the information you wrote down. When you've done that, use Chart 3 to rank these ten behaviors in order of importance to your child. In other words, on the first line you'll write down the behavior that you think is causing your child the *most* difficulty. Toward the bottom you'll write down the behaviors you think apply only slightly. If any of the ten do not apply at all, don't write them down. For example, if your child already eats a balanced, nourishing breakfast every day, don't write that one down. If your child has a problem behavior not included on your list of ten, add it whenever you think it fits in, according to its importance. But do record all behaviors which you think will require even a little change.

2: SUGGESTED WEIGHT CHARTS

My child's ideal weight: ————————————————

Suggested Weight By Height

Height (Inches)	Weight (Pounds)	Height (Inches)	Weight (Pounds)
20	8	40	35
22	10	42	39
24	13	44	42
26	16	46	46
28	19	48	51
30	22	50	55
32	25	52	61
34	27	54	68
36	28	56	75
38	32		

As children grow taller the weight differences between boys as a group and girls as a group become more pronounced.

Height (Inches)	Boys' Weight (Pounds)	Girls' Weight (Pounds)
58	103–117	95–107
60	110–127	100–115
62	118–136	106–122
64	124–144	114–130
66	132–152	122–138
68	140–160	129–148
70	148–170	138–157
72	156–178	144–164

SUGGESTED WEIGHT RANGE BY AGE

Age	Boys' Weight	Girls' Weight
1	20–24	18–23
2	25–30	23–28
3	29–35	27–33
4	33–40	31–40
5	37–45	35–44
6	42–48	39–47
7	46–55	44–54
8	50–62	50–62
9	55–68	56–72
10	62–78	64–83

Age	Boys' Weight	Girls' Weight
11	69–88	72–95
12	77–99	81–105
13	88–114	90–116
14	98–127	98–125
15	112–143	105–132
16	123–154	110–136

STEP 4: Choose the First Behavior to Change

As you now know, there are many reasons why your child is overweight. Your child didn't acquire his or her bad eating habits all at once, and it's sensible not to try to change them all at once, even though you may be tempted to do so. Doing this would upset the child and would be too hard to keep up; the result would most likely be the fate of most adults' diets: two weeks of unpleasant effort, followed by a return to the old patterns. Instead, you will choose one behavior to change, concentrate on that one for two weeks and then (while you keep up the first new behavior) add a second. You'll keep up the first two and two weeks later add a third, and so on until you've covered all of the problem behaviors. Gradually the new behaviors will become habits and will need very little attention from you. The entire effort will take about six months. That sounds like a long time and a lot of trouble. Only you can decide whether it's worth doing in order to give your child a lifetime of better health and

3: PROBLEM BEHAVIOR TO BE CHANGED

(1 = behavior most difficult to change; 10 = behavior least difficult to change.)

1. _____

2. _____

3. _____

4. _____

5. _____

6. _____

7. _____

8. _____

9. _____

10. _____

4: THE FIRST BEHAVIOR TO BE CHANGED

Description of Behavior: (including when it takes place, under what circumstances, etc.)

increased happiness. If you decide it is, choose the behavior at the very *bottom* of the list. "Now that you've
got me hooked, why can't I start at the top of the list?"
you may ask. Very simply because it's best to start with
the easily changed behaviors. In this endeavor as in others,
the child must learn to crawl before learning to walk. The
success you and your son or daughter experience in changing the least troublesome behaviors will give you the confidence and the motivation to keep going and eventually
change the most difficult behaviors. And concentrating on
one behavior for two weeks before adding another one
means that the first one will be well on its way to becoming a habit by the time you tackle a second one. Take
a moment now to fully describe on Chart 4 the first behavior that you want to change.

STEP 5: Decide Which Incentives to Use to Change This Behavior

At the top of Chart 5 jot down the first behavior you're
going to change. Then have another look at Chapter
Seven and choose an incentive that you feel will be useful
in changing this particular behavior and also write that
down, along with any details of how you're going to apply
it. Again, it is important that you actually write this down.
You'll refer to it during the next few months.

STEP 6: Carry Out the Behavior Change

For the next two weeks, you'll be concentrating only
on this one behavior. Since it's the least difficult one to

5: INCENTIVES TO USE

Behavior:

Incentive(s) to use:

How to apply these incentives:

change, you probably won't have any problems. If you do, you may have to find a more effective incentive or to break the behavior down into smaller steps. Try not to push too hard; if increasing your child's exercise is what you're working on, settle for a couple of extra walks to the store at first. You can then gradually increase the amount of exercise. If a behavior does involve several steps, concentrate on one step the first week, another the next, and delay the introduction of the next behavior by another week or even two if that seems sensible to you. Always be sensitive to your child's reactions, but on the other hand let resistance be your cue to change the plan a bit, not your cue to give up. The next step tells you how to keep track of your efforts and your child's progress.

STEP 7: Record Your Child's Weight and Your Efforts on the Calendar

Following this chapter there is a six-month calendar. Each week weigh your child twice, once on Monday, once on Thursday, and record those figures. Plot them on the weight charts at the end of the calendar. Write the starting weight on the line as indicated. Then complete the scale. For example, if the starting weight is 88 pounds, then write 88 on the line for starting weight and fill in the rest of the chart as shown in the example below. Put a dot on the chart each day that the weight is taken.

Eventually you'll see the line linking the dots moving downward. Typically, at some points the weight loss will stop for a while and then resume. Also, since you're attacking the least troublesome behaviors first, it may take a while for the weight loss to begin; right at first your child may even gain weight as his appetite control center tries to adjust its level. Don't worry about this, and don't let it trick you into trying to move more quickly. Follow your schedule and you will see results at a sensible, healthy pace.

At the beginning of each week jot down the behavior you'll be working on and the incentives you'll be using. Each day check whether you have paid attention to the behavior changes you are working on. At the bottom of each page you can make notes about any difficulties you're encountering or any adjustments you've had to make. Doing this only takes a minute at the end of the day, but acts as a reminder and motivator. Resolve to make it one of *your* new habits.

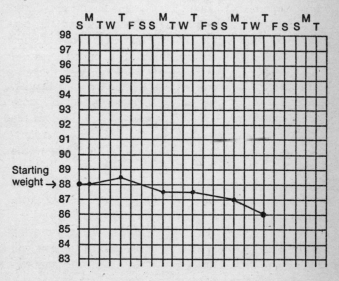

STEP 8: Continue This Pattern Until All the Behaviors Are Changed

Continue on the recommended schedule. You may slow it down if you feel that's a good idea, but don't try to speed it up. Be sure to keep on weighing your child and filling in the calendar forms. As was explained in the incentives chapter, after a while behaviors become habits, and then they no longer require special rewards. This is another reason for spacing out the behavior change; by the time you get around to the fourth behavior, you should be able to phase out the rewards for the first behavior.

If you ever begin to get discouraged by the effort, go back to reread Chapter Two. Remind yourself of the penalties your child has already endured and the ones yet to come if his or her obesity isn't corrected. And think ahead to the day—and we admit it may be some years off —when your son or daughter is mature enough to realize that all this trouble was in his or her best interests and comes up to you and says, "Thanks, Mom, thanks, Dad." If you follow through with your program, you can be sure that happy day will arrive.

MONTH _____

SUNDAY	Behavior for this week: Incentive for this week:
MONDAY	Child's weight: Did you follow your plan YES ☐ today? NO ☐
TUESDAY	Did you follow your plan YES ☐ today? NO ☐
WEDNESDAY	Did you follow your plan YES ☐ today? NO ☐
THURSDAY	Child's weight: Did you follow your plan YES ☐ today? NO ☐
FRIDAY	Did you follow your plan YES ☐ today? NO ☐
SATURDAY	Did you follow your plan YES ☐ today? NO ☐

NOTES

MONTH _____

SUNDAY	Behavior for this week: Incentive for this week:	
MONDAY	Child's weight: Did you follow your plan today?	YES ☐ NO ☐
TUESDAY	Did you follow your plan today?	YES ☐ NO ☐
WEDNESDAY	Did you follow your plan today?	YES ☐ NO ☐
THURSDAY	Child's weight: Did you follow your plan today?	YES ☐ NO ☐
FRIDAY	Did you follow your plan today?	YES ☐ NO ☐
SATURDAY	Did you follow your plan today?	YES ☐ NO ☐
NOTES		

MONTH _____

SUNDAY	Behavior for this week: Incentive for this week:	
MONDAY	Child's weight: Did you follow your plan today?	YES ☐ NO ☐
TUESDAY	Did you follow your plan today?	YES ☐ NO ☐
WEDNESDAY	Did you follow your plan today?	YES ☐ NO ☐
THURSDAY	Child's weight: Did you follow your plan today?	YES ☐ NO ☐
FRIDAY	Did you follow your plan today?	YES ☐ NO ☐
SATURDAY	Did you follow your plan today?	YES ☐ NO ☐
NOTES		

MONTH _____

SUNDAY	Behavior for this week: Incentive for this week:
MONDAY	Child's weight: Did you follow your plan today? YES □ NO □
TUESDAY	Did you follow your plan today? YES □ NO □
WEDNESDAY	Did you follow your plan today? YES □ NO □
THURSDAY	Child's weight: Did you follow your plan today? YES □ NO □
FRIDAY	Did you follow your plan today? YES □ NO □
SATURDAY	Did you follow your plan today? YES □ NO □
NOTES	

MONTH _____

SUNDAY	Behavior for this week: Incentive for this week:	
MONDAY	Child's weight: Did you follow your plan today?	YES ☐ NO ☐
TUESDAY	Did you follow your plan today?	YES ☐ NO ☐
WEDNESDAY	Did you follow your plan today?	YES ☐ NO ☐
THURSDAY	Child's weight: Did you follow your plan today?	YES ☐ NO ☐
FRIDAY	Did you follow your plan today?	YES ☐ NO ☐
SATURDAY	Did you follow your plan today?	YES ☐ NO ☐
NOTES		

MONTH _____

SUNDAY	Behavior for this week: Incentive for this week:	
MONDAY	Child's weight: Did you follow your plan today?	YES ☐ NO ☐
TUESDAY	Did you follow your plan today?	YES ☐ NO ☐
WEDNESDAY	Did you follow your plan today?	YES ☐ NO ☐
THURSDAY	Child's weight: Did you follow your plan today?	YES ☐ NO ☐
FRIDAY	Did you follow your plan today?	YES ☐ NO ☐
SATURDAY	Did you follow your plan today?	YES ☐ NO ☐
NOTES		

MONTH _____

SUNDAY	Behavior for this week: Incentive for this week:
MONDAY	Child's weight: Did you follow your plan today?　　YES ☐　NO ☐
TUESDAY	Did you follow your plan today?　　YES ☐　NO ☐
WEDNESDAY	Did you follow your plan today?　　YES ☐　NO ☐
THURSDAY	Child's weight: Did you follow your plan today?　　YES ☐　NO ☐
FRIDAY	Did you follow your plan today?　　YES ☐　NO ☐
SATURDAY	Did you follow your plan today?　　YES ☐　NO ☐
NOTES	

MONTH _____

SUNDAY	Behavior for this week: Incentive for this week:
MONDAY	Child's weight: Did you follow your plan today? YES ☐ NO ☐
TUESDAY	Did you follow your plan today? YES ☐ NO ☐
WEDNESDAY	Did you follow your plan today? YES ☐ NO ☐
THURSDAY	Child's weight: Did you follow your plan today? YES ☐ NO ☐
FRIDAY	Did you follow your plan today? YES ☐ NO ☐
SATURDAY	Did you follow your plan today? YES ☐ NO ☐
NOTES	

MONTH _____

SUNDAY	Behavior for this week: Incentive for this week:	
MONDAY	Child's weight: Did you follow your plan today?	YES ☐ NO ☐
TUESDAY	Did you follow your plan today?	YES ☐ NO ☐
WEDNESDAY	Did you follow your plan today?	YES ☐ NO ☐
THURSDAY	Child's weight: Did you follow your plan today?	YES ☐ NO ☐
FRIDAY	Did you follow your plan today?	YES ☐ NO ☐
SATURDAY	Did you follow your plan today?	YES ☐ NO ☐
NOTES		

MONTH _____

SUNDAY	Behavior for this week: Incentive for this week:	
MONDAY	Child's weight: Did you follow your plan today?	YES ☐ NO ☐
TUESDAY	Did you follow your plan today?	YES ☐ NO ☐
WEDNESDAY	Did you follow your plan today?	YES ☐ NO ☐
THURSDAY	Child's weight: Did you follow your plan today?	YES ☐ NO ☐
FRIDAY	Did you follow your plan today?	YES ☐ NO ☐
SATURDAY	Did you follow your plan today?	YES ☐ NO ☐
NOTES		

MONTH _____

SUNDAY	Behavior for this week: Incentive for this week:
MONDAY	Child's weight: Did you follow your plan today? YES ☐ NO ☐
TUESDAY	Did you follow your plan today? YES ☐ NO ☐
WEDNESDAY	Did you follow your plan today? YES ☐ NO ☐
THURSDAY	Child's weight: Did you follow your plan today? YES ☐ NO ☐
FRIDAY	Did you follow your plan today? YES ☐ NO ☐
SATURDAY	Did you follow your plan today? YES ☐ NO ☐

NOTES

MONTH _____

SUNDAY	Behavior for this week: Incentive for this week:	
MONDAY	Child's weight: Did you follow your plan today?	YES ☐ NO ☐
TUESDAY	Did you follow your plan today?	YES ☐ NO ☐
WEDNESDAY	Did you follow your plan today?	YES ☐ NO ☐
THURSDAY	Child's weight: Did you follow your plan today?	YES ☐ NO ☐
FRIDAY	Did you follow your plan today?	YES ☐ NO ☐
SATURDAY	Did you follow your plan today?	YES ☐ NO ☐
NOTES		

MONTH _____

SUNDAY	Behavior for this week: Incentive for this week:
MONDAY	Child's weight: Did you follow your plan today? YES ☐ NO ☐
TUESDAY	Did you follow your plan today? YES ☐ NO ☐
WEDNESDAY	Did you follow your plan today? YES ☐ NO ☐
THURSDAY	Child's weight: Did you follow your plan today? YES ☐ NO ☐
FRIDAY	Did you follow your plan today? YES ☐ NO ☐
SATURDAY	Did you follow your plan today? YES ☐ NO ☐
NOTES	

MONTH _____

SUNDAY	Behavior for this week: Incentive for this week:
MONDAY	Child's weight: Did you follow your plan today?　　YES ☐　NO ☐
TUESDAY	Did you follow your plan today?　　YES ☐　NO ☐
WEDNESDAY	Did you follow your plan today?　　YES ☐　NO ☐
THURSDAY	Child's weight: Did you follow your plan today?　　YES ☐　NO ☐
FRIDAY	Did you follow your plan today?　　YES ☐　NO ☐
SATURDAY	Did you follow your plan today?　　YES ☐　NO ☐
NOTES	

MONTH _____

SUNDAY	Behavior for this week: Incentive for this week:	
MONDAY	Child's weight: Did you follow your plan today?	YES ☐ NO ☐
TUESDAY	Did you follow your plan today?	YES ☐ NO ☐
WEDNESDAY	Did you follow your plan today?	YES ☐ NO ☐
THURSDAY	Child's weight: Did you follow your plan today?	YES ☐ NO ☐
FRIDAY	Did you follow your plan today?	YES ☐ NO ☐
SATURDAY	Did you follow your plan today?	YES ☐ NO ☐
NOTES		

MONTH _____

SUNDAY	Behavior for this week: Incentive for this week:	
MONDAY	Child's weight: Did you follow your plan today?	YES ☐ NO ☐
TUESDAY	Did you follow your plan today?	YES ☐ NO ☐
WEDNESDAY	Did you follow your plan today?	YES ☐ NO ☐
THURSDAY	Child's weight: Did you follow your plan today?	YES ☐ NO ☐
FRIDAY	Did you follow your plan today?	YES ☐ NO ☐
SATURDAY	Did you follow your plan today?	YES ☐ NO ☐
NOTES		

MONTH _____

SUNDAY	Behavior for this week: Incentive for this week:
MONDAY	Child's weight: Did you follow your plan today? YES ☐ NO ☐
TUESDAY	Did you follow your plan today? YES ☐ NO ☐
WEDNESDAY	Did you follow your plan today? YES ☐ NO ☐
THURSDAY	Child's weight: Did you follow your plan today? YES ☐ NO ☐
FRIDAY	Did you follow your plan today? YES ☐ NO ☐
SATURDAY	Did you follow your plan today? YES ☐ NO ☐
NOTES	

MONTH _____

SUNDAY	Behavior for this week: Incentive for this week:
MONDAY	Child's weight: Did you follow your plan today? YES ☐ NO ☐
TUESDAY	Did you follow your plan today? YES ☐ NO ☐
WEDNESDAY	Did you follow your plan today? YES ☐ NO ☐
THURSDAY	Child's weight: Did you follow your plan today? YES ☐ NO ☐
FRIDAY	Did you follow your plan today? YES ☐ NO ☐
SATURDAY	Did you follow your plan today? YES ☐ NO ☐
NOTES	

MONTH _____

SUNDAY	Behavior for this week: Incentive for this week:
MONDAY	Child's weight: Did you follow your plan today? YES ☐ NO ☐
TUESDAY	Did you follow your plan today? YES ☐ NO ☐
WEDNESDAY	Did you follow your plan today? YES ☐ NO ☐
THURSDAY	Child's weight: Did you follow your plan today? YES ☐ NO ☐
FRIDAY	Did you follow your plan today? YES ☐ NO ☐
SATURDAY	Did you follow your plan today? YES ☐ NO ☐
	NOTES

MONTH _____

SUNDAY	Behavior for this week: Incentive for this week:
MONDAY	Child's weight: Did you follow your plan today? YES ☐ NO ☐
TUESDAY	Did you follow your plan today? YES ☐ NO ☐
WEDNESDAY	Did you follow your plan today? YES ☐ NO ☐
THURSDAY	Child's weight: Did you follow your plan today? YES ☐ NO ☐
FRIDAY	Did you follow your plan today? YES ☐ NO ☐
SATURDAY	Did you follow your plan today? YES ☐ NO ☐
NOTES	

MONTH _____

SUNDAY	Behavior for this week:	
	Incentive for this week:	
MONDAY	Child's weight: Did you follow your plan today?	YES ☐ NO ☐
TUESDAY	Did you follow your plan today?	YES ☐ NO ☐
WEDNESDAY	Did you follow your plan today?	YES ☐ NO ☐
THURSDAY	Child's weight: Did you follow your plan today?	YES ☐ NO ☐
FRIDAY	Did you follow your plan today?	YES ☐ NO ☐
SATURDAY	Did you follow your plan today?	YES ☐ NO ☐
NOTES		

MONTH _____

SUNDAY	Behavior for this week: Incentive for this week:	
MONDAY	Child's weight: Did you follow your plan today?	YES ☐ NO ☐
TUESDAY	Did you follow your plan today?	YES ☐ NO ☐
WEDNESDAY	Did you follow your plan today?	YES ☐ NO ☐
THURSDAY	Child's weight: Did you follow your plan today?	YES ☐ NO ☐
FRIDAY	Did you follow your plan today?	YES ☐ NO ☐
SATURDAY	Did you follow your plan today?	YES ☐ NO ☐
NOTES		

MONTH _____

SUNDAY	Behavior for this week: Incentive for this week:
MONDAY	Child's weight: Did you follow your plan today? YES ☐ NO ☐
TUESDAY	Did you follow your plan today? YES ☐ NO ☐
WEDNESDAY	Did you follow your plan today? YES ☐ NO ☐
THURSDAY	Child's weight: Did you follow your plan today? YES ☐ NO ☐
FRIDAY	Did you follow your plan today? YES ☐ NO ☐
SATURDAY	Did you follow your plan today? YES ☐ NO ☐
NOTES	

MONTH _____

SUNDAY	Behavior for this week: Incentive for this week:	
MONDAY	Child's weight: Did you follow your plan today?	YES ☐ NO ☐
TUESDAY	Did you follow your plan today?	YES ☐ NO ☐
WEDNESDAY	Did you follow your plan today?	YES ☐ NO ☐
THURSDAY	Child's weight: Did you follow your plan today?	YES ☐ NO ☐
FRIDAY	Did you follow your plan today?	YES ☐ NO ☐
SATURDAY	Did you follow your plan today?	YES ☐ NO ☐
NOTES		

MONTH _____

SUNDAY	Behavior for this week: Incentive for this week:	
MONDAY	Child's weight: Did you follow your plan today?	YES ☐ NO ☐
TUESDAY	Did you follow your plan today?	YES ☐ NO ☐
WEDNESDAY	Did you follow your plan today?	YES ☐ NO ☐
THURSDAY	Child's weight: Did you follow your plan today?	YES ☐ NO ☐
FRIDAY	Did you follow your plan today?	YES ☐ NO ☐
SATURDAY	Did you follow your plan today?	YES ☐ NO ☐
NOTES		

MONTH _____

SUNDAY	Behavior for this week: Incentive for this week:
MONDAY	Child's weight: Did you follow your plan today? YES ☐ NO ☐
TUESDAY	Did you follow your plan today? YES ☐ NO ☐
WEDNESDAY	Did you follow your plan today? YES ☐ NO ☐
THURSDAY	Child's weight: Did you follow your plan today? YES ☐ NO ☐
FRIDAY	Did you follow your plan today? YES ☐ NO ☐
SATURDAY	Did you follow your plan today? YES ☐ NO ☐
NOTES	

MONTH _____

SUNDAY	Behavior for this week: Incentive for this week:
MONDAY	Child's weight: Did you follow your plan today?　　　YES ☐　NO ☐
TUESDAY	Did you follow your plan today?　　　YES ☐　NO ☐
WEDNESDAY	Did you follow your plan today?　　　YES ☐　NO ☐
THURSDAY	Child's weight: Did you follow your plan today?　　　YES ☐　NO ☐
FRIDAY	Did you follow your plan today?　　　YES ☐　NO ☐
SATURDAY	Did you follow your plan today?　　　YES ☐　NO ☐
NOTES	

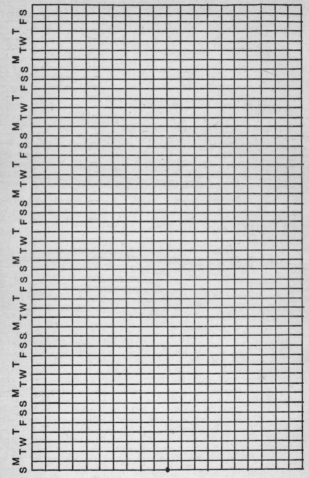

SIX-MONTH WEIGHT CHART

S M T W T F S S M T W T F S S M T W T F S S M T W T F S S M T W T F S S M T W T F S

Starting
weight →

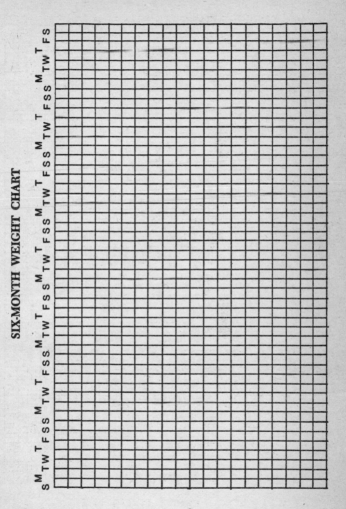

SIX-MONTH WEIGHT CHART

S M T W T F S S M T W T F S S M T W T F S S M T W T F S S M T W T F S S M T W T F S

Starting
weight →

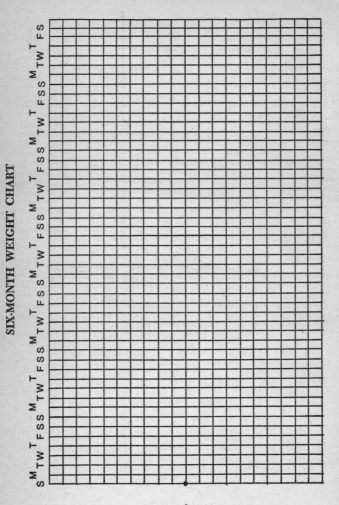

SIX-MONTH WEIGHT CHART

S M T W T F S S M T W T F S S M T W T F S S M T W T F S S M T W T F S S M T W T F S

Starting weight →

SIX-MONTH WEIGHT CHART

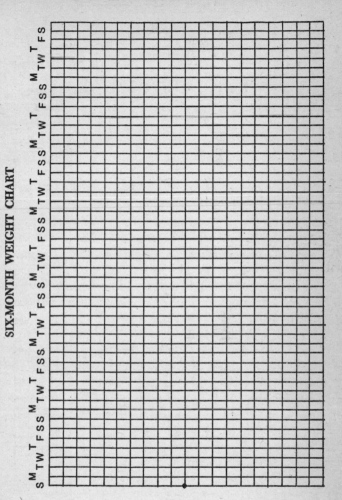

Starting
weight →

9

Keeping Off the Pounds

The Importance of Staying Slim

What should you do when your child has reached the point of no longer being overweight? It's a happy moment but also a dangerous one. As hard as it is to do, many people succeed in losing weight. However, very few succeed in hanging on to their new-found slimness. They slowly go back to their old weaknesses and once again begin to add pounds. Eventually they find they're right back where they started. Then they must not only confront their flabby bodies, they must also confront themselves with another failure. The approach we have described in this book makes this sort of failure less likely because it emphasizes long-term changes in basic eating habits. Even so, there are some things you can do to guarantee that your child continues his or her success. We'll describe these things now, and we suggest you reread this chapter periodically once your child has achieved his or her goal weight.

Avoiding the Food Trap

It's easy to fall into the trap of thinking that once your child is no longer overweight it wouldn't hurt to have snack foods in the house again. But having lots of ice cream, candy, pastries, and other sugar-laden foods available threatens to undo the new behavior patterns you have so carefully instilled. The most important thing to remember is that your child's weight will always be determined by food intake and by the amount of energy used up. It's no good thinking, "Well, now that Bobby is slim, a few snacks won't hurt." They *will* hurt, and although the weight gain may be quite slow, just as the weight loss was quite slow, it *will* take place. You will come under special pressure during certain holidays. At Halloween, children come home with bags full of junk food; often, enough to destroy their diets for the following month or two. Make a practice of giving out fruit and small trinkets instead of candy and encourage your friends to do the same. Don't deny your children the pleasure of dressing up and going from door to door if they want to, but agree beforehand upon something they'll get as a "treat" from you, in exchange for handing over for disposal the candy they collect. Thanksgiving and Christmas are associated in people's minds with good eating, but good eating doesn't have to mean filling up until you're ready to burst. By all means, take the time to fix delicious and elaborate meals as a way of celebrating, but when planning the menu consider the calories and choose light desserts.

You know the kinds of eating behaviors that led your child to be overweight. You also know he or she is learning to have better control of eating. But your child still needs your help to keep temptation away. Keep the situation manageable for your child, even during holidays and other special occasions.

Rewarding Success

Gradually you have phased out rewards for specific behaviors that have now become habits. You should now switch to celebrating periods of successful weight-maintenance. You can even schedule your celebrations ahead of time and color in the dates on your calendar. The celebration can take any form you like: It may just be a half hour when you praise your child and give him or her a lot of attention, or you may use one of the incentives you've previously found successful (for example, taking the child to the movies). Have frequent celebrations at first, then spread them out over longer intervals. The first two might be weekly, the next two every two weeks, and then monthly. These events remind the child (and you) that it's important to keep up good eating habits, and they continue to build the child's self-esteem. Naturally you will have to allow for some weight gain as part of the growth process. To estimate how much weight will be gained due to growth from year to year, refer back to the "ideal weight" chart on pages 129 – 131.

Recording Weight after the Goal Has Been Reached

Your child is now used to being weighed twice a week and having his or her behavior recorded on a chart. Continue to do this as an "early warning system" to alert you to weight gains. While a younger child may simply forget to weigh himself, or herself, once in a while, teenagers (and adults too) may avoid weighing themselves if they know they've been straying from the path of sensible eating. They know the scales will soon reflect an unwanted weight gain. By keeping up the twice-weekly weighing process you'll be helping your child to avoid falling back into poor eating habits.

The Life-Long Exercise Habit

Exercise continues to bring benefits long after the goal weight has been reached. Appearance continues to improve and vitality and energy continue to increase as the level of exercise increases. Thus you should continue to encourage and reward the kinds of exercise that can become a life-long habit. As we discussed in Chapter Six, the best kind of exercise is noncompetitive and can be done alone, such as swimming, bike-riding, and jogging. All of these can gradually be increased; for example, your child may slowly build up daily jogging until he or she reaches 1 or 2 or even 3 or 4 miles per day. As a result, your child will have greater energy reserves, better tolerance of stress, and greater self-confidence. Once these benefits begin to become obvious to your child, the exercise provides its own built-in motivation to continue and increase it.

Appealing to Your Child's Pride

A child may continue to think of himself or herself as fat even after reaching goal weight. Children who have been grossly overweight for most of their lives may continue to lumber along, rather than walk, and to hold their arms away from their sides as if to accommodate imaginary rolls of fat. With this sort of attitude, the desire to continue good eating habits may grow weak. The child's psychological condition must be helped to catch up with his or her physical condition. It will take time, but new clothes and a new hair style are one way to assist the change. They are visible to your child and his or her friends, who are more likely to respond to handsome new clothes than to a gradual weight loss. The resulting compliments will help build up the child's self-confidence and ability to see himself or herself in a new light.

Avoiding Showdowns

What you have done is take control of your child's eating behavior. You will want to give this control to your child gradually. How quickly a child can assume major responsibility for eating behavior is determined partly by age, partly by past success. It's possible, and probably necessary, for you to take almost complete control of your child's eating behavior at home, especially during the preteen years. As your child grows older, parental control becomes more difficult. In the teen years, as self-assertion and independence become more important to children, control of food can be a struggle. If food becomes the objective of a battle for control, the teenager may demonstrate independence by breaking food rules.

The safest way to proceed is to avoid making food the object of a showdown. Don't link other criticisms to what you think of your teenager's eating habits. For example, don't say something like, "I'm getting sick of seeing your room in a mess and of seeing you stuff yourself with candy bars!" During your child's period of rebellion, it's best to work silently. Do serve balanced meals at home and don't buy snacks. Appeal to your teenager's desire for social acceptance, for example by casually rewarding a weight loss with some money for a new dress or jacket. If your child suffers from acne and consults a dermatologist, ask the doctor beforehand to discuss the possible connection between diet and skin problems. If your teenager has an adult he or she respects, perhaps a teacher, an aunt or an uncle, or a family friend, that person may be willing to have a heart-to-heart talk with your teenager about losing weight. The key is for you, as the parent, to avoid becoming too closely identified with this issue if your child is in the rebellion phase of adolescence. Otherwise your child may gorge himself or herself, in the belief that gaining more weight would be a way of getting back at you. The immature young adult is capable of doing this without stopping to think of the disastrous consequences it will have for himself or herself.

Dealing with Setbacks

The best way to deal with setbacks is to prepare for them. A setback may last for a minute or a day or a year, depending upon what you decide—yes, you can *decide* how long it will last. It's a poor decision to tell yourself that all is lost because your child goes on an eating binge. Let's see what causes sudden lapses in good eating habits.

A child may start thinking about "forbidden" foods as he or she approaches the goal weight. It may almost become an obsession, and the child may want to reward himself or herself for good behavior by cramming down lots of candy and ice cream. From a strictly logical viewpoint this would be compared to a drowning man who slowly and laboriously pulls himself out of the sea, and then celebrates by jumping back in! However, we're dealing with emotion, not with logic. You probably can't prevent your child from going on a binge if he or she is determined to have one. Afterward, you can't undo it with punishment.

There's another factor at work. The famous Harvard physiologist Jean Meyer has written at length about the tendency of the body to maintain the status quo. When it loses weight there seems to be a tendency to gain it back again. This drive is less powerful if the weight loss has been slow, which is one reason why we have suggested a gradual change in your child's habits. But even so, your child may experience a period of feeling especially hungry once the goal weight has been reached, and the temptation to respond is great.

Finally, stress and anxiety can play a destructive role, too, especially in the case of the overweight teenager. An overweight high school girl, for example, may decide that her social problems stem from the fact that she's fat. When she slims down, she expects an immediate improvement in her social life, and if it doesn't happen, she may figure that good eating habits are a fraud. She may even go back to being overweight because it gives her an excuse for lack of social success. Although being slim has lots of benefits, it's not a cure-all. The newly trim person will still have to learn all the social graces, and it can be especially difficult if obesity has made him or her shy in the past.

Whatever the reason for the child's loss of control, the parent can help by being supportive and constructive. In the case of the teenage girl, the parents could point out that a good physical appearance is just one aspect of social success, and encourage her to recognize that all of her friends are going through some difficulties dealing with adolescence. In the case of the child who rewards himself by eating too much, the parents can point out that continued overeating leads back to the "Hey kid, how come you're so fat?" situation, and can put special emphasis on rewarding periods of weight maintenance. In all cases, the parent can sit down with the child, discuss the reasons for the binge, and ask the child to make a decision about how long he or she wants to continue to abandon control of his or her behavior. The consequences of losing control should be discussed, too—a week-long binge could require two months of careful control to right the balance while the damage of a short spree in a candy shop could be undone in a couple of days. Discussing the issue in this way helps to remove it from the sphere of the purely emotional. Most youngsters will choose to regain control immediately and will be able to do so. Even if they don't, they experience a real choice and understand the consequences of their decision, which makes it more likely they will be able to resist such binges in the future.

Conclusion

There's not much more to say, except—Congratulations! By the time your child has reached goal weight, you'll have had to solve some problems and make a sustained effort. Maybe you thought you wouldn't be able to keep it up. Maybe you even gave up for a little while and then started again. Your reward is knowing your child is free of the penalties of being overweight. People don't usually ask, "Hey kid, how come you're so slim, and healthy, and happy?" If someone *does* ask your child that question, take a bow!

Chapter Summary

Losing excess weight is only half the battle. Keeping it off is the other half. Parents can help by continuing to bar the door to snack and junk foods, even during the holidays and other special occasions. Rewards continue to have a place once extra weight is gone. The rewards now are used to celebrate periods of successful weight maintenance. Exercise also continues to be important and to bring increasing benefits during this period. Despite your best efforts, there will be setbacks from time to time. The way to deal with this is to expect the setbacks, be supportive and constructive when your child loses control, and have your child decide how long the out-of-control period will be. You can help motivate your child to maintain the right weight level by continuing the twice-weekly weighings and by appealing to your child's pride in his or her appearance. With teenagers, it may be necessary to play down your desire to control their behavior, otherwise they may choose to overeat as a way of rebelling against you.

Appendix A
Calorie Content of Common Foods

Food and approximate measure		Food Energy (Calories)
EGGS		
Eggs, large, 24 ounces per dozen:		
Raw:		
Whole, without shell	1 egg	75
White of egg	1 white	15
Yolk of egg	1 yolk	60
Cooked:		
Boiled, shell removed	2 eggs	160
Scrambled with milk and fat	1 egg	110
FATS, OILS		
Butter and margarine, 4 sticks per pound:		
Sticks, 2	1 cup	1625
Stick, 1/8	1 tablespoon	100
Pat or square (64 per pound)	1 pat	50
Fats, cooking:		
Lard	1 cup	1985

Food and approximate measure		Food Energy (Calories)
Lard	1 tablespoon	125
Vegetable fats	1 cup	1770
Vegetable fats	1 tablespoon	110
Oils, salad or cooking:		
Corn	1 tablespoon	125
Cottonseed	1 tablespoon	125
Olive	1 tablespoon	125
Soybean	1 tablespoon	125
Salad dressings:		
Blue cheese	1 tablespoon	80
Commercial, mayonnaise type	1 tablespoon	65
French	1 tablespoon	60
Home-cooked, boiled	1 tablespoon	30
Mayonnaise	1 tablespoon	110
Thousand Island	1 tablespoon	75

FRUITS AND FRUIT PRODUCTS

Measure and weight apply to entire vegetable or fruit including parts not usually eaten.

Apple juice, bottled or canned	1 cup	120
Applesauce, canned:		
Sweetened	1 cup	230
Unsweetened or artificially sweetened	1 cup	100
Apples, raw, 2-1/2 inch diameter, about 3 per pound	1 apple	70
Apple brown betty	1 cup	345

Food and approximate measure		Food Energy (Calories)

FRUITS AND FRUIT PRODUCTS

Applesauce and apricots, canned, strained, or junior (baby food)	1 ounce	25
Apricots:		
Raw, about 12 per pound	3 apricots	55
Canned in heavy syrup:		
Halves and syrup	1 cup	220
Halves (medium) and syrup	4 halves; 2 tablespoons syrup	105
Dried:		
Uncooked, 40 halves, small	1 cup	390
Cooked, unsweetened, fruit and liquid	1 cup	240
Apricot nectar, canned	1 cup	140
Avocados, raw:		
California varieties, mainly Fuerte:		
10-ounce avocado, about 3-1/2 by 4-1/4 inches, peeled and pitted	1/2 avocado	185
1/2 inch cubes	1 cup	260
Florida varieties:		
13-ounce avocado, about 4 by 3 inches, peeled and pitted	1/2 avocado	160
1/2 inch cubes	1 cup	195

Food and approximate measure		Food Energy (Calories)
Bananas, raw, 6 by 1-1/2 inches, about 3 per pound	1 banana	85
Blackberries, raw	1 cup	85
Blueberries, raw	1 cup	85
Cantaloupes, raw; medium, 5 inch diameter, about 1-2/3 pounds	1/2 melon	60
Cherries:		
Raw, sweet, with stems	1 cup	80
Canned, red, sour, pitted, heavy syrup	1 cup	230
Cranberry juice cocktail, canned	1 cup	160
Cranberry sauce, sweetened, canned, strained	1 cup	405
Dates, domestic, natural, and dry, pitted, cut	1 cup	490
Figs:		
Raw, small, 1-1/2 inch diameter, about 12 per pound	3 figs	90
Dried, large, 2 by 1 inch	1 fig	60
Fruit cocktail, canned in heavy syrup, solids and liquid	1 cup	195
Grapefruit:		
Raw, medium, 4-1/2 inch diameter:		
White	1/2 grapefruit	55
Pink or red	1/2 grapefruit	60
Raw sections, white	1 cup	75

Food and approximate measure		Food Energy (Calories)

FRUITS AND FRUIT PRODUCTS

Canned, white:

| Syrup pack, solids & liquid | 1 cup | 175 |
| water pack, solids & liquid | 1 cup | 70 |

Grapefruit juice:

| Fresh | 1 cup | 95 |

Canned, white:

| Unsweetened | 1 cup | 100 |
| Sweetened | 1 cup | 130 |

Frozen, concentrate, unsweetened

| Undiluted, can, 6 ounces | 1 can | 300 |
| Diluted with 3 parts water | 1 cup | 100 |

Frozen, concentrate, sweetened:

| Undiluted, can, 6 ounces | 1 can | 350 |
| Diluted with 3 parts water | 1 cup | 115 |

Dehydrated:

| Crystals, can, 4 ounces | 1 can | 430 |
| Prepared with water (1 pound yields about 1 gallon) | 1 cup | 100 |

Grapes, raw:

American type (slip skin) such as Concord, Delaware, Niagara, Catawba, and Scuppernong — 1 cup — 65

European types (adherent skin), such as Malaga,

Food and approximate measure		Food Energy (Calories)
Muscat, Thompson Seedless, Emperor, and Flame Tokay	1 cup	95
Grape juice, bottled or canned	1 cup	165
Lemons, raw, medium, 2-1/4 inch diameter	1 lemon	20
Lemon juice:		
Fresh	1 cup	60
	1 tablespoon	5
Canned, unsweetened	1 cup	55
Lemonade concentrate, frozen, sweetened:		
Undiluted, can, 6 fluid ounces	1 can	430
Diluted with 4-1/3 parts water	1 cup	110
Lime juice:		
Fresh	1 cup	65
Canned	1 cup	65
Limeade concentrate, frozen, sweetened:		
Undiluted, can, 6 fluid ounces	1 can	410
Diluted with 4-1/3 parts water	1 cup	105
Oranges, raw:		
California, Navel (winter), 2-4/5 inch diameter	1 orange	60
Florida, all varieties, 3 inch diameter	1 orange	75
Orange juice:		
Fresh, Valencia (summer) California	1 cup	115

Food and approximate measure		Food Energy (Calories)
FRUITS AND FRUIT PRODUCTS		
Florida varieties:		
Early and midseason	1 cup	100
Late season, Valencia	1 cup	110
Canned, unsweetened	1 cup	120
Frozen concentrate:		
Undiluted can, 6 ounces	1 can	330
Diluted with 3 parts water	1 cup	110
Dehydrated:		
Crystals, can, 4 ounces	1 can	430
Prepared with water (1 pound yields about 1 gallon)	1 cup	115
Orange and grapefruit juice:		
Frozen concentrate:		
Undiluted, can, 6 ounces	1 can	325
Diluted with 3 parts water	1 cup	110
Papayas, raw, 1/2 inch cubes	1 cup	70
Peaches:		
Raw:		
Whole, medium, 2 inch diameter, about 4 per pound	1 peach	35
sliced	1 cup	65
Canned, yellow-fleshed solids and liquid:		
Syrup pack, heavy:		
Halves or slices	1 cup	200

Food and approximate measure		Food Energy (Calories)
Halves and syrup	2 halves and 2 tablespoons syrup	90
Water pack	1 cup	75
Strained or chopped (baby food)	1 ounce	25
Dried:		
Uncooked	1 cup	420
Cooked, unsweetened, 10 to 12 halves & 6 tablespoons liquid	1 cup	220
Frozen:		
Carton, 12 ounce, not thawed	1 carton	300
Can, 16 ounce, not thawed	1 can	400
Peach nectar, canned	1 cup	120
Pears:		
Raw, 3 by 2-1/2 inch diameter	1 pear	100
Canned, solids and liquid:		
Syrup pack, heavy:		
Halves or slices	1 cup	195
Halves and syrup	2 halves and 2 tablespoons syrup	90
Water pack	1 cup	80
Strained or chopped (baby food)	1 ounce	20

Food and approximate measure		Food Energy (Calories)

FRUITS AND FRUIT PRODUCTS

Food and approximate measure		Food Energy (Calories)
Pear nectar, canned	1 cup	130
Persimmons, Japanese or Kaki, raw, seedless, 2-1/2 inch diameter	1 persimmon	75
Pineapple:		
Raw, diced	1 cup	75
Canned, heavy syrup pack, Solids and liquid:		
Crushed	1 cup	195
Slices, with juice	2 small or 1 large and 2 tablespoons juice	90
Pineapple juice, canned	1 cup	135
Plums (except prunes):		
Raw, 2 inch diameter, 2 ounce	1 plum	25
Canned, syrup pack (Italian prunes):		
Plums, with pits and juice	1 cup	205
Plums, without pits and juice	3 plums, 2 tablespoons juice	100
Prunes, dried "softenized":		
Uncooked	4 prunes	70
Cooked, unsweetened, 17 to 18 prunes and 1/3 cup of liquid	1 cup	295

Food and approximate measure		Food Energy (Calories)
Prunes with tapioca, canned, strained, or junior (baby food)	1 ounce	25
Prune juice, canned	1 cup	200
Raisins, dried	1 cup	460
Raspberries, red:		
Raw	1 cup	70
Frozen, 10 ounce not thawed	1 carton	275
Rhubarb, cooked, sugar added	1 cup	385
Strawberries:		
Raw, capped	1 cup	55
Frozen, 10 ounce not thawed	1 carton	310
Frozen, 16 ounce can, not thawed	1 can	495
Tangerines, raw, 2-1/2 inch dia. about 4 per pound	1 tangerine	40
Tangerine juice:		
Canned, unsweetened	1 cup	105
Frozen concentrate:		
Undiluted, can, 6 ounce	1 can	340
Diluted, 3 parts water	1 cup	115
Watermelon, raw, wedge 4 by 8 inches	1 wedge	115

GRAIN PRODUCTS

Barley, pearled, light, uncooked	1 cup	710
Biscuits, baking powder with enriched flour, 2-1/2 inch diameter	1 biscuit	140

Food and approximate measure		Food Energy (Calories)

GRAIN PRODUCTS

Bran flakes (40 percent bran), added thiamine	1 ounce	85
Breads:		
Boston brown bread, slice, 3 by 3/4 inches	1 slice	100
Cracked-wheat bread:		
Loaf, 1 pound, 20 slices	1 loaf	1190
Slice	1 slice	60
French or Vienna bread:		
Enriched, 1 pound loaf	1 loaf	1315
Unenriched, 1 pound loaf	1 loaf	1315
Italian bread:		
Enriched, 1 pound loaf	1 loaf	1250
Unenriched, 1 pound loaf	1 loaf	1250
Raisin bread:		
Loaf, 1 pound, 20 slices	1 loaf	1190
Slice	1 slice	60
Rye bread:		
American, light (1/3 rye, 2/3 wheat):		
Loaf, 1 pound, 20 slices	1 loaf	1100
Slice	1 slice	55
Pumpernickel, loaf, 1 pound	1 loaf	1115
White bread, enriched:		
1 to 2 percent nonfat dry milk°		
Loaf, 1 pound, 20 slices	1 loaf	1225
Slice	1 slice	60

Food and approximate measure		Food Energy (Calories)
3 to 4 percent nonfat dry milk:*		
Loaf, 1 pound	1 loaf	1225
Slice, 20 per loaf	1 slice	60
Slice, toasted	1 slice	60
Slice, 26 per loaf	1 slice	45
White bread, unenriched:		
1 to 2 percent nonfat dry milk:*		
Loaf, 1 pound, 20 slices	1 loaf	1225
Slice	1 slice	60
3 to 4 percent nonfat dry milk:*		
Loaf, 1 pound	1 loaf	1225
Slice, 20 per loaf	1 slice	60
Slice, toasted	1 slice	60
Slice, 26 per loaf	1 slice	45
5 to 6 percent nonfat dry milk:*		
Loaf, 1 pound, 20 slices	1 loaf	1245
Slice	1 slice	65
Wholewheat bread, made with		
2 percent nonfat dry milk:		
Loaf, 1 pound, 20 slices	1 loaf	1105
Slice	1 slice	55
Slice, toasted	1 slice	55
Breadcrumbs, dry, grated	1 cup	345

* When the amount of nonfat dry milk in commercial white bread is unknown, values for bread with 3 to 4 percent nonfat dry milk are suggested.

Food and approximate measure		Food Energy (Calories)

GRAIN PRODUCTS
Cakes:**

Angelfood cake, 2 inch piece	1 piece	110
Chocolate cake, 2 inch piece, chocolate icing	1 piece	445
Fruitcake, dark, enriched flour; piece 2 by 1/2 inch	1 piece	115
Gingerbread, enriched flour; piece 2 by 2 by 2 inches	1 piece	175
Plain cake and cupcakes, without icing:		
Piece, 3 by 2 by 1-1/2 inches	1 piece	200
Cupcake, 2-3/4 inch diameter	1 cupcake	145
Plain cake and cupcakes with chocolate icing:		
Sector, 2-inch	1 sector	370
Cupcake, 2-3/4 inch diameter	1 cupcake	185
Poundcake, old-fashioned (equal weights flour, sugar, fat, eggs):		
Slice 2-3/4 by 3 by 5/8 inches	1 slice	140
Sponge cake; sector, 2 inch	1 sector	120
Cookies:		
Plain and assorted, 3 inch diameter	1 cookie	120
Fig bars, small	1 fig bar	55

** Unenriched cake flour and vegetable cooking fat used unless otherwise specified.

Food and approximate measure		Food Energy (Calories)
Corn, rice, and wheat flakes, mixed, added nutrients	1 ounce	110
Corn flakes, added nutrients:		
Plain	1 ounce	110
Sugar-covered	1 ounce	110
Corn grits, degermed, cooked:		
Enriched	1 cup	120
Unenriched	1 cup	120
Cornmeal, white or yellow, dry:		
Whole ground, unbolted	1 cup	420
Degermed, enriched	1 cup	525
Corn muffins, enriched, de-germed cornmeal and enriched flour; muffin, 2-3/4 inch diameter	1 muffin	150
Corn, puffed, presweetened, added nutrients	1 ounce	110
Corn, shredded, added nutrients	1 ounce	110
Crackers:		
Graham, plain	4 small or 2 medium	55
Saltines, 2 inch square	2 crackers	35
Soda:		
Cracker, 2-1/2 inch square	2 crackers	50
Oyster crackers	10 crackers	45
Cracker meal	1 tablespoon	45
Doughnuts, cake-type	1 doughnut	125
Farina, regular, enriched, cooked	1 cup	100

Food and approximate measure		Food Energy (Calories)
GRAIN PRODUCTS		
Macaroni, cooked:		
Enriched:		
Cooked, firm stage (8 to 10 minutes; undergoes additional cooking in a food mixture)	1 cup	190
Cooked until tender	1 cup	155
Unenriched:		
Cooked, firm stage (8 to 10 minutes; undergoes additional cooking in a food mixture)	1 cup	190
Cooked until tender	1 cup	155
Macaroni (enriched) and cheese, baked	1 cup	470
Muffins, enriched white flour; muffin, 2-3/4 inch diameter	1 muffin	140
Noodles (egg noodles), cooked:		
Enriched	1 cup	200
Unenriched	1 cup	200
Oats (with or without corn), puffed, added nutrients	1 ounce	115
Oatmeal or rolled oats, regular or quick cooking, cooked	1 cup	130
Pancakes, 4 inch diameter:		
Wheat, enriched flour (home recipe)	1 cake	60

Food and approximate measure		Food Energy (Calories)
Buckwheat (mix, made with egg and milk)	1 cake	55
Piecrust, plain, baked:		
Enriched flour:		
Lower crust, 9 inch shell	1 crust	675
Double crust, 9 inch pie	1 double crust	1350
Unenriched flour:		
Lower crust, 9 inch shell	1 crust	675
Double crust, 9 inch pie	1 double crust	1350
Pies (piecrusts made with unenriched flour); sector, 4 inch:		
Apple	1 sector	345
Cherry	1 sector	355
Custard	1 sector	280
Lemon meringue	1 sector	305
Mince	1 sector	365
Pumpkin	1 sector	275
Pizza (cheese), 5-1/2 inch sector	1 sector	185
Popcorn, popped, oil and salt	1 cup	65
Pretzels, small stick	5 sticks	20
Rice, white (fully milled or polished), enriched, cooked:		
Common commercial varieties, all types	1 cup	185
Long grain, parboiled	1 cup	185
Rice, puffed, added nutrients, without salt	1 cup	55
Rice flakes, added nutrients	1 cup	115

Food and approximate measure		Food Energy (Calories)

GRAIN PRODUCTS
Rolls:
  Plain, pan; 12 per 16 ounce:

Enriched	1 roll	115
Unenriched	1 roll	115
Hard, round, 12 per 22 ounce	1 roll	160
Sweet, pan; 12 per 18 ounce	1 roll	135
Rye wafers, whole-grain, 2 by 3-1/2 inches	2 wafers	45

Spaghetti:
  Cooked, tender stage:

Enriched	1 cup	155
Unenriched	1 cup	155
Spaghetti with meat balls in tomato sauce (homemade)	1 cup	335
Spaghetti in tomato sauce with cheese (homemade)	1 cup	260
Waffles, enriched flour, 4-1/2 by 5-1/2 by 1/2 inch	1 waffle	210

Wheat, puffed:

With added nutrients (without salt)	1 ounce	105
With added nutrients, with sugar and honey	1 ounce	105
Wheat, rolled; cooked	1 cup	175
Wheat, shredded, plain (long, round, or bite-size)	1 ounce	100
Wheat and malted barley flakes, with added nutrients	1 ounce	110

Food and approximate measure		Food Energy (Calories)
Wheat flakes with added nutrients	1 ounce	100
Wheat flours:		
Wholewheat, from hard wheats	1 cup	400
All-purpose or family flour:		
Enriched, sifted	1 cup	400
Unenriched, sifted	1 cup	400
Self-rising, enriched	1 cup	385
Cake or pastry flour, sifted	1 cup	365
Wheat germ, crude, commercially milled	1 cup	245

MATURE DRY BEANS AND PEAS, NUTS, PEANUTS: RELATED PRODUCTS

Almonds, shelled	1 cup	850
Beans, dry:		
Common varieties, such as Great Northern, Navy, etc. canned:		
Red	1 cup	230
White with tomato sauce:		
With pork	1 cup	320
Without pork	1 cup	310
Lima, cooked	1 cup	260
Brazil nuts	1 cup	915
Cashew nuts, roasted	1 cup	760

Food and approximate measure		Food Energy (Calories)

MATURE DRY BEANS AND PEAS, NUTS, PEANUTS: RELATED PRODUCTS

Coconut:		
Fresh, shredded	1 cup	335
Dried, shredded, sweetened	1 cup	340
Cowpeas or blackeyed peas, dry,		
cooked	1 cup	190
Peanuts, roasted, salted:		
Halves	1 cup	840
Chopped	1 tablespoon	55
Peanut butter	1 tablespoon	95
Peas, split, dry, cooked	1 cup	290
Pecans:		
Halves	1 cup	740
Chopped	1 tablespoon	50
Walnuts, shelled:		
Black or native, chopped	1 cup	790
English or Persian:		
Halves	1 cup	650
Chopped	1 tablespoon	50

MEAT, POULTRY, FISH, SHELLFISH: RELATED PRODUCTS

Trimmed to retail basis: Outer layer of fat on the cut was removed to within approximately 1/2 inch of the lean. Deposits of fat within the cut not removed.

Bacon, broiled or fried, crisp	2 slices	100

Food and approximate measure		Food Energy (Calories)
Beef, trimmed to retail basis, cooked:		
Cuts braised, simmered, or pot-roasted:		
Lean and fat	3 ounces	245
Lean only	2.5 ounces	140
Hamburger (ground beef) broiled:		
Lean	3 ounces	185
Regular	3 ounces	245
Roast, oven-cooked, no liquid added:		
Relatively fat, such as rib:		
Lean and fat	3 ounces	375
Lean only	1.8 ounces	125
Relatively lean, such as round:		
Lean and fat	3 ounces	165
Lean only	2.7 ounces	125
Steak, broiled:		
Relatively fat, such as sirloin:		
Lean and fat	3 ounces	330
Lean only	2 ounces	115
Relatively lean, such as round:		
Lean and fat	3 ounces	220
Lean only	2.4 ounces	130

Food and approximate measure		Food Energy (Calories)

MEAT, POULTRY, FISH,
SHELLFISH: RELATED
PRODUCTS

Beef, canned:		
Corned beef	3 ounces	185
Corned beef hash	2 ounces	155
Beef, dried and chipped	2 ounces	115
Beef and vegetable stew	1 cup	210
Beef pot pie, baked; individual pie, 4-1/4 inch diameter, weight before baking about 8 ounces	1 pie	560
Chicken, cooked:		
Flesh only, broiled	3 ounces	115
Breast, fried, 1/2 breast:		
With bone	3.3 ounces	155
Flesh and skin only	2.7 ounces	155
Drumstick, fried:		
With bone	2.1 ounces	90
Flesh and skin only	1.3 ounces	90
Chicken, canned, boneless	3 ounces	170
Chicken pot pie. See Poultry pot pie.		
Chile con carne, canned:		
With beans	1 cup	335
Without beans	1 cup	510
Heart, beef, lean, braised	3 ounces	160

Food and approximate measure		Food Energy (Calories)
Lamb, trimmed to retail basis, cooked:		
Chop, thick, with bone, broiled	1 chop, 4.8 ounces	400
Lean and fat	4 ounces	400
Lean only	2.6 ounces	140
Leg, roasted:		
Lean and fat	3 ounces	235
Lean only	2.5 ounces	130
Shoulder, roasted:		
Lean and fat	3 ounces	285
Lean only	2.3 ounces	130
Liver, beef, fried	2 ounces	130
Pork, cured, cooked:		
Ham, light cure, lean and fat, roasted	3 ounces	245
Luncheon meat:		
Boiled ham, sliced	2 ounces	135
Canned, spiced or unspiced	2 ounces	165
Pork, fresh, trimmed to retail basis, cooked:		
Chop, thick with bone	1 chop, 3.5 ounces	260
Lean and fat	2.3 ounces	260
Lean only	1.7 ounces	130
Roast, oven-cooked, no liquid added:		
Lean and fat	3 ounces	310

Food and approximate measure		Food Energy (Calories)

MEAT, POULTRY, FISH, SHELLFISH: RELATED PRODUCTS

Food and approximate measure		Food Energy (Calories)
Lean only	2.4 ounces	175
Cuts, simmered:		
Lean and fat	3 ounces	320
Lean only	2.2 ounces	135
Poultry pot pie, individual pie, 4-1/2 inch diameter, weight before baking about 8 ounces	1 pie	535
Sausage:		
Bologna, sliced, 4.1 by 0.1 inch	8 slices	690
Frankfurter, cooked	1 frankfurter	155
Pork, links or patty cooked	4 ounces	540
Tongue, beef, braised	3 ounces	210
Turkey pot pie. See Poultry pot pie.		
Veal, cooked:		
Cutlet, without bone, broiled	3 ounces	185
Roast, medium, fat, medium done; lean and fat	3 ounces	230
Fish and Shellfish:		
Bluefish, baked or broiled	3 ounces	135
Clams:		
Raw, meat only	3 ounces	65
Canned, solids and liquids	3 ounces	45
Crabmeat, canned	3 ounces	85

Food and approximate measure		Food Energy (Calories)
Fish sticks, breaded, cooked, frozen; stick, 3.8 by 1.0 by 0.5 inch	10 sticks or 8 ounce pkg.	400
Haddock, fried	3 ounces	140
Mackerel:		
Broiled, Atlantic	3 ounces	200
Canned, Pacific, solids and liquid	3 ounces	155
Ocean perch, breaded (egg and breadcrumbs), fried	3 ounces	195
Oysters, meat only:		
Raw, 13–19 medium selects	1 cup	160
Oyster stew, 1 part oysters to 3 parts milk, 3 to 4 oysters	1 cup	200
Salmon, pink, canned	3 ounces	120
Sardines, Atlantic, canned in oil, drained solids	3 ounces	175
Shad, baked	3 ounces	170
Shrimp, canned, meat only	3 ounces	100
Swordfish, broiled with butter or margarine	3 ounces	150
Tuna, canned in oil, drained solids	3 ounces	170

Food and approximate measure		Food Energy (Calories)

MILK, CREAM, CHEESE:
RELATED PRODUCTS
Milk, cow's:

Fluid, whole (3.5 percent fat)	1 cup	160
Fluid, nonfat (skim)	1 cup	90
Buttermilk, cultured, from skim milk	1 cup	90
Evaporated, unsweetened, undiluted	1 cup	345
Condensed, sweetened, undiluted	1 cup	980
Dry, whole	1 cup	515
Dry, nonfat, instant	1 cup	250

Milk, goat's:

Fluid, whole	1 cup	165

Cream:

Half-and-half (cream & milk)	1 cup	325
	1 tablespoon	20
Light, coffee or table	1 cup	505
	1 tablespoon	30
Whipping, unwhipped (volume about double when whipped):		
Light	1 cup	715
	1 tablespoon	45
Heavy	1 cup	840
	1 tablespoon	55

Food and approximate measure		Food Energy (Calories)
Cheese:		
Blue or Roquefort type	1 ounce	105
Cheddar or American:		
Ungrated	1 inch cube	70
Grated	1 cup	445
	1 tablespoon	30
Cheese:		
Cheddar, process	1 ounce	105
Cheese foods, Cheddar	1 ounce	90
Cottage cheese, from skim milk:		
Creamed	1 cup	240
	1 ounce	30
Uncreamed	1 cup	195
	1 ounce	25
Cream cheese	1 ounce	105
	1 tablespoon	55
Swiss (domestic)	1 ounce	105
Milk beverages:		
Cocoa	1 cup	235
Chocolate-flavored milk drink (made with skim milk)	1 cup	190
Malted milk	1 cup	280
Milk desserts:		
Cornstarch pudding, plain	1 cup	276
Custard, baked	1 cup	285

Food and approximate measure		Food Energy (Calories)

MILK, CREAM, CHEESE:
RELATED PRODUCTS

Ice cream, plain, factory packed:		
Slice or cut brick, 1/8 of quart brick	1 slice	145
Container	3-1/2 fluid ounces	130
Container	8 fluid ounces	295
Ice milk	1 cup	285
Yogurt, from partially skimmed milk	1 cup	120

SUGAR, SWEETS

Candy:		
Caramels	1 ounce	115
Chocolate, milk, plain	1 ounce	150
Fudge, plain	1 ounce	115
Hard candy	1 ounce	110
Marshmallows	1 ounce	90
Chocolate syrup, thin type	1 tablespoon	50
Honey, strained or extracted	1 tablespoon	65
Jams and preserves	1 tablespoon	55
Jellies	1 tablespoon	55
Molasses, cane:		
Light (first extraction)	1 tablespoon	50
Blackstrap (third extraction)	1 tablespoon	45

Food and approximate measure		Food Energy (Calories)
Syrup, table blends (chiefly corn, light and dark)	1 tablespoon	60
Sugars (cane or beet):		
Granulated	1 cup	770
	1 tablespoon	45
Lump, 1-1/8 by 3/4 by 3/8 inch	1 lump	25
Powdered, stirred before measuring	1 cup	495
	1 tablespoon	30
Brown, firm-packed	1 cup	820
	1 tablespoon	50

VEGETABLES AND VEGETABLE PRODUCTS

Asparagus:		
Cooked, cut spears	1 cup	35
Canned spears, medium:		
Green	6 spears	20
Bleached	6 spears	20
Beans:		
Lima, immature, cooked	1 cup	180
Snap, green:		
Cooked:		
In small amount of water, short time	1 cup	30
In large amount of water, long time	1 cup	30

Food and approximate measure		Food Energy (Calories)

VEGETABLES AND VEGETABLE PRODUCTS

Canned:		
Solids and liquid	1 cup	45
Strained or chopped (baby food)	1 ounce	5
Bean sprouts. See Sprouts.		
Beets, cooked, diced	1 cup	50
Broccoli spears, cooked	1 cup	40
Brussels sprouts, cooked	1 cup	45
Cabbage:		
Raw:		
Finely shredded	1 cup	25
Coleslaw	1 cup	120
Cooked:		
In small amount of water, short time	1 cup	35
In large amount of water, long time	1 cup	30
Cabbage, celery or Chinese:		
Raw, leaves and stalk, 1 inch pieces	1 cup	15
Cabbage, spoon (or bokchoy), cooked	1 cup	20
Carrots:		
Raw:		
Whole, 5-1/2 inch by 1 inch	1 carrot	20
Grated	1 cup	45
Cooked, diced	1 cup	45

Food and approximate measure		Food Energy (Calories)
Canned, strained or chopped (baby food)	1 ounce	10
Cauliflower, cooked, flower buds	1 cup	25
Celery, raw:		
Stalk, large outer, 8 by about 1-1/2 inches at root end	1 stalk	5
Pieces, diced	1 cup	15
Collards, cooked	1 cup	55
Corn, sweet:		
Cooked, ear 5 by 3/4 inches*	1 ear	70
Canned, solids and liquid	1 cup	170
Cowpeas, cooked, immature seeds	1 cup	175
Cucumbers, 10 ounce, 7-1/2 by 2 inches		
Raw, pared	1 cucumber	30
Raw, pared, center slice 1/8 inch thick	6 slices	5
Dandelion greens, cooked	1 cup	60
Endive, curly (including escarole)	2 ounces	10
Kale, leaves and stems, cooked	1 cup	30
Lettuce, raw:		
Butterhead, as Boston types; head, 4 inch diameter	1 head	30
Crisp, as Iceberg; head, 4-3/4 inch diameter	1 head	60

* Measure and weight apply to entire vegetable or fruit including parts not usually eaten.

		Food Energy (Calories)
Food and approximate measure		
VEGETABLES AND VEGETABLE PRODUCTS		
Looseleaf, or bunching varieties, leaves	2 large	10
Mushrooms, canned, solids and liquid	1 cup	40
Mustard greens, cooked	1 cup	35
Okra, cooked, pod, 3 by 5/8 inch	8 pods	25
Onions:		
Mature:		
Raw, onions 2-1/2 inch diameter	1 onion	40
Cooked	1 cup	60
Young green, small without tops	6 onions	20
Parsley, raw, chopped	1 tablespoon	1
Parsnips, cooked	1 cup	100
Peas, green:		
Cooked	1 cup	115
Canned, solids and liquid	1 cup	165
Canned, strained (baby food)	1 ounce	15
Peppers, hot, red, without seeds, dried (ground chili powder, added seasonings)	1 tablespoon	50
Peppers, sweet:		
Raw, medium, about 6 per pound:		
Green pod without stems and seeds	1 pod	15

Food and approximate measure		Food Energy (Calories)
Red pod without stems and seeds	1 pod	20
Canned pimientos, medium	1 pod	10
Potatoes, medium (3 per pound, raw):		
Baked, peeled after baking	1 potato	90
Boiled:		
Peeled after boiling	1 potato	105
Peeled before boiling	1 potato	80
French-fried, piece 2 by 1/2 by 1/2 inch:		
Cooked in deep fat	10 pieces	155
Frozen, heated	10 pieces	125
Mashed:		
Milk added	1 cup	125
Milk and butter added	1 cup	185
Potato chips, medium, 2 inch diameter	10 chips	115
Pumpkin, canned	1 cup	75
Radishes, raw, small	4 radishes	5
Sauerkraut, canned, solids and liquid	1 cup	45
Spinach:		
Cooked	1 cup	40
Canned, drained solids	1 cup	45
Canned, strained or chopped (baby food)	1 ounce	10

Food and approximate measure		Food Energy (Calories)

VEGETABLES AND VEGETABLE PRODUCTS

Sprouts, raw:		
Mung bean	1 cup	30
Soybean	1 cup	40
Squash:		
Cooked:		
Summer, diced	1 cup	30
Winter, baked, mashed	1 cup	130
Canned, winter, strained and chopped (baby food)	1 ounce	10
Sweet potatoes:		
Cooked, medium, 5 by 2 inches, weight raw about 6 ounces		
Baked, peeled after baking	1 sweet potato	155
Boiled, peeled after boiling	1 sweet potato	170
Candied, 3-1/2 by 2-1/4 inches	1 sweet potato	295
Canned, vacuum or solid pack	1 cup	235
Tomatoes:		
Raw, medium, 2 by 2-1/2 inches, about 3 per pound	1 tomato	35
Canned	1 cup	50
Tomato juice, canned	1 cup	45
Tomato catsup	1 tablespoon	15
Turnips, cooked, diced	1 cup	35

Food and approximate measure		Food Energy (Calories)
Turnip greens:		
Cooked:		
In small amount of water, short time	1 cup	30
In large amount of water, long time	1 cup	25
Canned, solids and liquid	1 cup	40

MISCELLANEOUS ITEMS

Beer (average 3.6 percent alcohol)	1 cup	100
Beverages, carbonated:		
Cola type	1 cup	95
Ginger ale	1 cup	70
Bouillon cube, 5/8 inch	1 cube	5
Chili powders. See Vegetables, peppers.		
Chili sauce (mainly tomatoes)	1 tablespoon	20
Chocolate:		
Bitter or baking	1 ounce	145
Sweet	1 ounce	150
Cider. See Fruits, apple juice		
Gelatin, dry:		
Plain	1 tablespoon	35
Dessert powder, 3 ounce package	1/2 cup	315
Gelatin dessert, ready-to-eat:		
Plain	1 cup	140
With fruit	1 cup	160

Food and approximate measure		Food Energy (Calories)

MISCELLANEOUS ITEMS

Olives, pickled:

Green	4 medium or	
	3 extra large	
	or 2 giant	15
Ripe	3 small or	
	2 large	15

Pickles, cucumber:

Dill, large, 4 by 1-3/4 inch	1 pickle	15
Sweet, 2-3/4 by 3/4 inch	1 pickle	30
Popcorn. See Grain Products		
Sherbet, orange	1 cup	260

Soups, canned; ready-to-serve (prepared with equal volume of water):

Bean with pork	1 cup	170
Beef noodle	1 cup	70
Beef bouillon, broth, consomme	1 cup	30
Chicken noodle	1 cup	65
Clam chowder	1 cup	85
Cream soup (mushroom)	1 cup	135
Minestrone	1 cup	105
Pea, green	1 cup	130
Tomato	1 cup	90
Vegetable with beef broth	1 cup	80
Starch (cornstarch)	1 cup	465
	1 tablespoon	30

Food and approximate measure		Food Energy (Calories)
Tapioca, quick-cooking, granulated, dry, stirred before measuring	1 cup	535
	1 tablespoon	35
Vinegar	1 tablespoon	2
White sauce, medium	1 cup	430
Yeast:		
Baker's		
Compressed	1 ounce	25
Dry active	1 ounce	80
Yeast:		
Brewer's dry, debittered	1 tablespoon	25
Yogurt. See Milk, cream, cheese, related products.		

Appendix B
Healthful Snack Recipes

As was discussed earlier in the book, snacks often destroy the nutritional balance of a child's diet and overload it with calories. Your long-term goal should be to eliminate snacks altogether. A short-term remedy is to substitute healthful snacks for candy bars, chocolates, and ice cream. Here are the characteristics of a healthful snack:

it is low in calories

it doesn't contain much sugar

it's not so filling that it will destroy the child's appetite

it has nutritional value

Using these criteria, you can come up with your own snack ideas, but in this appendix we present a few of ours.

Nature's Own Preparations

Nature provides her own recipes for delicious, ready-to-eat foods. They contain no unnatural preservatives and no refined sugar, and they are "convenience" foods in the truest sense of the word: all you do is remove the package (the peel or shell), if necessary, and eat. The first category is *vegetables*, especially:

carrots   celery   radishes   tomatoes   cucumbers

The tomatoes can be eaten just as you'd eat an apple; the others can be washed, cut, and kept on a plate in the refrigerator.

The second group of such foods is made up of *fruits* and *berries*, especially:

apples	cherries
oranges	grapes
grapefruit	plums
bananas	tangerines
apricots	watermelon
pears	cantaloupe
peaches	strawberries and raspberries
pineapple	blueberries and blackberries

If you buy these foods when they're in season, they need not be too expensive. Even out of season, seldom is a piece of fruit as expensive, ounce for ounce, as chocolate or a candy bar. If fresh fruit isn't available, you may buy it canned, but be sure it is packed in its own juice, not in syrup.

The last group of foods under this heading is *nuts*. These are nutritious, but they also tend to be high in calories and so should be eaten in limited quantities. It's best to buy the nuts still in their shells—having to crack the shells and extract the nutmeat slows down the eating process. Recommended are:

English walnuts and black walnuts   pecans

peanuts   almonds   chestnuts

Initially your children may not be too keen on these natural snacks. But if you have lots of them around and at the same time phase out the cupcakes, swiss rolls, ice cream, and candy bars, your youngsters will make the transition.

Liquids

Soda pop is another culprit that contributes to overweight and also rots teeth. We suggest you substitute:

fruit juices   vegetable juices   milk   water

We include water because it is essential for digestion and for the efficient working of the kidneys. Also, it provides valuable minerals. Be careful to distinguish between fruit juices and fruit drinks. The latter often are nothing more than sweetened and artificially flavored water, lacking the nutritional value of fruit juices.

Salads

Many households have abandoned the habit of serving a salad with lunch and dinner. If that's the case in your house, you should consider offering small salads as snacks. Even children who don't care for cooked vegetables often do like the crunchiness of raw vegetables. Don't limit your salads to lettuce and tomatoes; you can also chop up and add cucumbers, green onions, radishes, green peppers, leeks, celery, cabbage, and many other vegetables. Also, don't forget that fruit salads are particularly welcome in the summer. Below, we offer recipes for two unusual salads:

SALAD SANDWICH

1 7 ounce can of tuna
1/2 teaspoon crushed oregano leaves
1/4 teaspoon salt
a dash of pepper
1/4 cup of low-calorie mayonnaise
1 loaf French or Italian bread
1 small onion
1 red pepper
1 cup shredded lettuce

Drain and flake the tuna and mix in the oregano leaves, salt, pepper, and mayonnaise. Cut the loaf of bread lengthwise, almost to the end. Lift up the top half, and fill the bottom half with the tuna mixture, then add slices of green and red pepper, onion, and lettuce. Close the loaf and cut into snack-size segments.

RAVISHING ROOT

1 dozen radishes
2 tablespoons chives, chopped
2 tablespoons nonfat powdered milk
2 tablespoons parsley, chopped
1 tablespoon water

Mix chives and parsley in powdered milk and stir in the water. Roll the mixture into tiny balls (it's easier if you wet your hands first). Cut the radishes in half and place one ball on each half radish.

Soups

A hot soup can make a good snack, especially on cool days. Broths are relatively low in calories and you can make them yourself with meat or chicken stock. Most of us find it too time consuming to make other kinds of soup from scratch, especially since such a variety of canned soups are available. But here's a recipe for a recommended soup that's quickly made:

HOMEMADE CHEESE SOUP

1 cup condensed skim milk
1-1/2 cups cottage cheese
1 teaspoon curry power
1/4 teaspoon salt
1/8 teaspoon pepper
1 tablespoon chives

Very slowly add the milk and the cottage cheese into a blender. Run the blender at high speed after each additional small amount is added. Add the curry, salt, and pepper and mix. Cook in a saucepan over medium heat for 5 minutes. Sprinkle the chives on top.

Bread and Sandwiches

Earlier, we suggested that you serve wholewheat bread rather than white bread. You might also consider making your own bread and experiment with different kinds. Here's our recipe for corn bread:

CORN BREAD

1 cup flour (unsifted)
1 cup corn meal
4 teaspoons baking powder
1/2 teaspoon salt
1 cup skim milk
2 eggs
1/3 cup margarine

Mix the flour, corn meal, baking powder, and salt in a large bowl. Blend in the eggs, milk, and margarine and beat for one minute. Use a greased 8-inch (square) baking pan and bake at 425 degrees until done (20 to 25 minutes).

There are an almost infinite number of sandwiches. Here's one that's tasty; cut into small pieces, it makes a snack for several people. In larger quantity, it makes a main course meal:

PUMPERNICKEL TUNA SANDWICH

Pumpernickel bread (3–4 slices)
Raw tomato
Lettuce
4 eggs
1 small can tuna (7 ounce)
2 tablespoons chopped parsley
1 tablespoon margarine
1 tablespoon grated onion
a dash of pepper

Mix the tuna, onion, pepper, parsley, and eggs. Melt the margarine in a medium-sized skillet and pour in the above mixture. Cook over medium-low heat till set, stirring occasionally. Put a lettuce leaf and tomato slice on each slice of bread, and pour the hot mixture over the top.

Finally, here's a meatless variation of the Ruben sandwich:

BEEFLESS RUBEN

1 slice toast
1/4 teaspoon caraway seeds
3/4 tablespoon prepared mustard
1 slice Swiss cheese
1/2 cup sauerkraut (drained)

Spread the mustard on the toast and sprinkle on the caraway seeds. Add the cheese slice and put the sauerkraut on
tip. Broil until the top is lightly browned.

Your own cookbook will offer other snack recipes, but
again we stress that snacks shouldn't play too big a role
in your child's diet. Your ingenuity and skill as a cook is
much better invested in providing balanced meals. This
includes hearty breakfasts. If your children aren't used
to eating any breakfast, ease them into the habit with the
following recipe:

QUICK MIX

1/2 cup skim milk
1 or 2 slices whole-grain bread
1/2 cup orange juice
1 egg
1 teaspoon lemon juice

Simply mix all the ingredients for two or three minutes in
a blender.

We finish up with an alternative recipe for that breakfast favorite, pancakes. These are delicious just as they
are, so don't let your children drown them in syrup. If

they do want a topping, try fruit yogurt, thinned with a
bit of milk.

2 cups unsifted flour
1/4 cup corn oil
3 teaspoons baking powder
1 teaspoon salt
1-3/4 cups skim milk
2 teaspoons honey
2 eggs

In a large bowl, mix the flour, baking powder, salt, and
honey. Add the milk, corn oil, and eggs. Mix well. Cook
on a hot griddle. When the pancake is bubbly and the
edges are dry, turn it over. The batter can also be used to
make waffles with a waffle iron.